HIV/AIDS and agriculture in sub-Saharan Africa

HIV/AIDS and agriculture in sub-Saharan Africa

Impact on farming systems, agricultural
practices and rural livelihoods –
An overview and annotated bibliography

AWLAE SERIES No. 1

Tanja R. Müller
Wageningen University

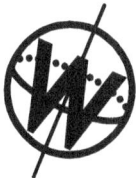

Wageningen Academic
P u b l i s h e r s

CIP-data Koninklijke Bibliotheek Den Haag

ISBN 9076998469

Subject headings:
HIV/AIDS impact
rural livelihoods
gender and food security

First published, 2004

Foto cover:
Stefan Boness – IPON

Wageningen Academic Publishers

The Netherlands, 2004

Printed in The Netherlands

Abstract

This publication is the first in a three part series looking at HIV/AIDS and agriculture in sub-Saharan Africa, with the overall objective of providing a resource base on the most crucial issues to consider when looking at rural development in sub-Saharan Africa in a broad sense in the times of HIV/AIDS. It describes the impact of the epidemic as it has emerged over the last decades at different levels of the agricultural sector, namely the farming system level, the livelihood level, and the household level. In a further step, less well researched impacts on the agricultural estate sector as well as pastoralism are discussed. One overarching issue that emerges is the importance of gender attributes to adequately understand and address HIV/AIDS impact on agricultural production systems in general and household food security in particular - the topic at the centre of the second part of the series. The text ends with a discussion of HIV/AIDS in relation to other shocks that befall rural livelihoods and a call for more holistic research approaches that integrate famine and other disaster literatures with HIV/AIDS impact studies. It is followed by an annotated bibliography.

Table of contents

Preface

This publication is the first in a three part series being produced within the context of the AWLAE Programme based at Wageningen University and Research Centre (WUR). AWLAE stands for African Women Leaders in Agriculture and the Environment, a pan-African non-governmental organisation (NGO) founded by Winrock International and based in Nairobi, Kenya.

The AWLAE Programme in Wageningen is funded by the Dutch Ministry of Foreign Affairs (DGIS) as a research and training programme in scientific and leadership skills. Within its parameters, 20 African women from 12 different countries come to Wageningen for their doctoral degree (PhD) in the period 2002 to 2007. The 12 participating countries cover much of Africa's regional diversity. They include from eastern Africa Uganda, Tanzania, Kenya and Ethiopia; from southern Africa Zimbabwe and South Africa; and from western Africa Nigeria, Ghana, Senegal, Benin, Mali and Côte d'Ivoire. The project leader is Dr. Julia Gitobu who is based in the AWLAE office in Nairobi. At WUR, the chair group of Sociology of Consumers and Households manages the project and chairs the Academic Advisory Committee (for more information see http://www.socialsciences.wur.nl/sch).

The overall theme of the AWLAE Programme is twofold: the role of women in food systems in rural sub-Saharan Africa on one hand, combined with the impact of HIV/AIDS on food and livelihood systems on the other. Having said that, however, the actual research topics of the PhD candidates are rather diverse, comprising not only a focus on agricultural technologies to increase rural women's capacity for food production, processing and marketing, but equally such issues as the potential role of micro-finance institutions to empower women, questions of access to education for rural girls versus boys, and the role of rural women as care-givers - to name just a few examples. What makes the AWLAE project quite unique are the two cross-cutting themes all research projects have to locate themselves within: the impacts of HIV/AIDS within a particular research setting, and an emphasis on women's agency and possibilities for its enhancement.

The body of knowledge being produced within the different PhD research projects will greatly contribute to a better understanding of how different HIV/AIDS epidemics within and between countries and regions - stretching from eastern and southern Africa to western Africa - impact on diverse rural livelihoods and ultimately regional and national options for rural development. As such, it will bring together Anglophone and Francophone research findings and discourses which to this day often rarely take notice of each other, with the ultimate objective of increased networking and sharing of experiences among the various geographical settings.

Additionally, in looking at issues of wider rural development in relation to HIV/AIDS through the lens of implications for women's agency, more gender conscious policies are hoped to emerge in the future. Given the gendered nature of agricultural livelihoods, combined with the gendered impacts of HIV/AIDS, female scholars in particular can provide relevant policy analysis. In a further step, technically trained women armed with appropriate PhDs can help to bridge the gap between research and policy change.

This publication is the first in a series of three, with the overall objective of providing a resource base on the most crucial issues to consider when looking at rural development in sub-Saharan Africa in a broad sense in the times of HIV/AIDS. This first publication deals with the impact of HIV/AIDS on the agricultural sector. The second publication will explore the linkages between gender and HIV/AIDS, with a concrete focus on rural women and their role in food security and care giving. The third publication will discuss the HIV/AIDS epidemic as a wider development issue, as well as focus on agriculture-based mitigation strategies. All three publications comprise two parts: an essay outlining the major issues and summarizing research carried out to date, followed by an annotated bibliography introducing the most relevant literature (with a focus on literature that can be obtained within or from the Netherlands). Taken together, this publication series is meant to serve the wider academic community as well as development practitioners, the latter including national and multinational bodies as well as NGOs engaged in development assistance projects. It is intended in particular for PhD students and other researchers who work in settings were HIV/AIDS is a crucial factor in rural development and the welfare of rural households.

Lastly, it is hoped that this series helps to contribute to acknowledging the HIV/AIDS pandemic as at present the major challenge to human development in sub-Saharan Africa and beyond. At the same time - in accordance with the objectives of the AWLAE Programme - it is meant to give renewed impetus to the need to strengthens women's agency if the promises of human development are to be achieved and the fight against the epidemic is to be won eventually.

Anke Niehof
Chair AWLAE Academic Advisory Committee
Sociology of Consumers and Households Group (SCH) - WUR

List of acronyms

AIDS (SIDA)	Acquired Immune Deficiency Syndrome
AWLAE	African Women Leaders in Agriculture and the Environment
DFID	UK Department for International Development
DGIS	Dutch Ministry for Foreign Affairs
EQUINET	Regional Network for Equity in Health in Southern Africa
FANR	Food, Agriculture and Natural Resources
FAO	United Nations Food and Agricultural Organisation
FES	Friedrich Ebert Foundation
FSVM	Farming System Vulnerability Mapping
HHRAA	Health and Human Resources Analysis for Africa
HIV (VIH)	Human Immunodeficiency Virus
IAEN	International AIDS Economics Network
IFAD	International Fund for Agricultural Development
IFPRI	International Food Policy Research Institute
ISS	Institute of Social Studies The Hague
KIT	Royal Tropical Institute Amsterdam
LVM	Livelihood Vulnerability Mapping
MoA	Ministry of Agriculture
NAADS	National Agricultural Advisory Service Uganda
NGO	Non-Governmental Organisation
ODI	Overseas Development Institute London
PhD	Doctor of Philosophy
PRSP	Poverty Reduction Strategy Paper
RENEWAL	Regional Network on HIV/AIDS, Rural Livelihoods and Food Security in sub-Saharan Africa
ROAPE	Review of African Political Economy
SARA	Support for Analysis and Research in Africa
SASC	Southern African Development Community
UNAIDS	Joint United Nations Programme on HIV/AIDS
UNDP	United Nations Development Programme
UNRISD	United Nations Research Institute for Social Development
USAID	US Agency for International Development

WB	World Bank
WHO	World Health Organisation
WUR	Wageningen University and Research Centre

Key concepts

Susceptibility:	the chances of an individual becoming infected with the HIV virus
Vulnerability:	the likelihood of significant physical, social or economic impact occurring at individual, household, community or farm system level
Resistance:	ability of an individual to avoid infection
Resilience:	active response of infected persons that enables them to avoid the worst impacts of AIDS at different levels, or to recover to a level accepted as normal
Incidence:	number of new occurrences (infections) in a specified period of time, usually one calendar year
Prevalence:	pool of all infections at a given point in time

Categorisation of households

Afflicted household:	household in which one or more members is/are either ill or has/have died of AIDS related causes
Affected household:	household in which household members are not infected themselves, but have been affected by HIV/AIDS through for example the diversion of household resources to support an AIDS-afflicted household, the death of an extended family member who was contributing to the household, or orphans joining the household.

Unaffected household: household in which no member is ill or has died from AIDS related diseases, and which has not been affected by the illness or death of a member of any related household (such households are usually rare in high prevalence areas)

This categorisation was first made by Barnett & Blaikie (1992) and has since been used in a number of studies. The concept of 'afflicted household' has at times been criticised in that it may divert attention away from the systemic impact of the epidemic. This criticism has given way to a simple distinction between affected and unaffected households, whereby affected households include what is here distinguished as 'afflicted' and 'affected'. While much of the more recent literature follows this twofold categorisation, within this publication series the threefold distinction is used (only in the annotated bibliography 'affected household' is at times solely used if done so in the document discussed). Even though no detailed studies exist in which impact is strictly differentiated according to whether a household is afflicted or affected in the above defined sense, a distinction between the two is regarded as analytically useful in order to allow for the possibilities of difference in impact and mitigation strategies.

Part 1 – Overview

1. Introduction

When studying the social and economic impact of HIV/AIDS in the context of sub-Saharan Africa, one of the most important areas to consider is how the epidemic affects agriculture and rural livelihoods. This is the case for a number of reasons, some of the most prominent of which are the following:

Firstly, while HIV prevalence rates are generally higher in urban areas, the absolute number of people living with HIV is likely to be greater in rural areas, not least because over two thirds of the population is rural in most sub-Saharan countries (du Guerny, 2002; Topouzis, 1998). In addition, infection rates in rural areas are hard to measure and more prone to under-reporting and misdiagnosis, and the incidence of HIV/AIDS within rural households and communities can be difficult to detect. It has for example been observed that while distress sales of assets in the case of famine are highly visible affairs, with livestock being brought to market in high numbers, the selling of such assets in the case of AIDS is a rather low-key and subtle affair (Rugalema, 1999). Taken together, all these factors contribute to the fact that rural HIV remains to different extents invisible (Topouzis, 1998).

Secondly, there is a tendency within the private sector to shift the burden of AIDS by withdrawing sickness benefits, a move that often leads to an increased burden on rural households, as migrant workers may return to the rural areas once they fall ill. In addition, urban households have been reported to send AIDS orphans back to their 'home' village. As a result, the rural economy is bearing a large share of the cost of the epidemic while at the same time the possibility to call upon support from the urban economy is diminishing (de Waal, 2003).

Thirdly, in macro-economic terms, the countries most affected by HIV/AIDS are those most heavily reliant on agriculture, with the agricultural sector accounting for a significant portion of production as well as employing the majority of workers (Topouzis, 2000). In addition, (subsistence) agriculture remains an important component of the livelihoods of the majority of poor individuals who live in these countries (Haddad & Gillespie, 2001a). The impact of the epidemic on rural communities and economies, as well as on the agricultural sector as a whole, is thus of critical significance to such countries (Topouzis, 1998; 2000).[1]

This state of affairs also suggests that agriculture clearly has an important role to play in preventing and mitigating the effects of the epidemics.[2] But before its is possible to arrive at strategies for agricultural interventions, the impact of the epidemic on different parts of the agricultural sector needs to be understood in detail. Looking at this impact, two broad levels of analysis have been distinguished in the literature: the farming system level, and the farm-household system level (du Guerny, 2002).[3]

Within the systems' hierarchy, HIV/AIDS is first experienced at the farm-household system level, as it is first and foremost human beings who are infected, fall ill and eventually die. The epidemic then progresses through the system, potentially reaching and altering farming systems as well as wider regional and national systems (Barnett & Haslwimmer, 1995).

Impact at the farm-household system level of analysis has been studied either as (a) impact (on agricultural practices) at household level, including impact within households - the latter including issues such

---

[1] A study carried out in Kenya and discussed by Topouzis (2000) does additionally suggest that, relative to other sectors such as industry and services, the agricultural sector is disproportionally more severely affected by the epidemic. A similar line of thought is advanced by de Waal & Tumushabe (2003), who argue that the structure of especially the smallholder agricultural subsector is such that it is much less able to absorb the impacts of human labour losses associated with the epidemic than other sectors. More concrete evidence is needed to sustain this assertion.

[2] The plural 'epidemics' seems appropriate here, as indeed, there are many different HIV/AIDS epidemics, each with its own dynamics. In sub-Saharan Africa, these include epidemics fuelled by rural-urban links; epidemics among high risk groups (truck drivers, prostitutes); epidemics in rural areas fuelled by migration and so forth (see du Guerny, 2002). Agricultural interventions are appropriate only for some of these.

[3] A farm-household system generally consists of the following three sub-systems: the household as decision making unit; the farm and its crop and livestock activities; and the off-farm component (employment and income generating activities) - for further discussion see Barnett & Haslwimmer (1995).

as the distribution of nutritious food between boys and girls; and changes in entitlements to food, to land, to inheritance between senior and junior as well as between male and female household members; or as (b) impact at the level of (rural) livelihoods.

While both impacts are related with each other, they are not the same: Impact studies at household level look at the shock(s) individual households experience when one or more household members fall ill from HIV/AIDS related diseases and/or eventually die, and how the household responds to these shock(s). Whereas to look at HIV/AIDS as a livelihood shock includes a focus on how assets at community level become depleted, eventually leading to a livelihood crisis experienced in one way or another by the majority of households within a given community.

In a further step, whole farming systems might change due to the epidemic, particularly so in high prevalence areas - even though evidence which points to HIV/AIDS as the main cause for such changes is difficult to find, as other factors might have equally contributed to such changes, like for example changing weather patterns, increased livelihood diversification, changes in export crop markets, structural adjustment programmes, civil strive, or other shocks that befall rural livelihoods.

From the above it seems that what is required is to study HIV/AIDS impact at these three different levels - the household level, the livelihood level, and the farming system level - and put the findings of such studies in relation to each other. The first detailed field study carried out in Uganda in 1989 (Barnett & Blaikie, 1992) for example demonstrated that even in a robust and on the face of it not very vulnerable farming system such as that of Southern Uganda - with good soils, sufficient rainfall and a range of different crops - high levels of infection were even at that relatively early stage having an impact in terms of lowering levels of life in many rural households. Thus, indicators at household level can inform interventions at the farming system level, while at the same time an observed change in a particular farming system may mean that already a very high number of households are destitute.

The importance of looking at impact at all three levels of analysis and combine the results of such studies is due to the fact that (a) precise impact of the epidemic varies from place to place; (b) responses might need to be farming system or livelihood specific; (c) HIV/AIDS does not merely affect some agricultural subsectoral components, while leaving others unaffected; in contrast, if one component of the system is affected, it is likely that others will be so too, be it directly or indirectly - in other words, the impact of HIV/AIDS is systemic, thus the linkages between subsectors, institutions, and households need to be identified; and (d) it is important to downstream and upstream responses.

Overall, one needs to keep in mind that while it is possible to make general statements about implications of HIV/AIDS on farming systems, agricultural production, rural livelihoods, and household food security and well-being, responses must be developed in relation to specific situations - specific in terms of farming systems, geographical factors, and cultural factors. It has for example been shown that such simple issues as whether women are culturally allowed to ride bicycles can make a big difference at household level in terms of marketing agricultural produce when a male member dies. Other aspects to be considered are whether societies or communities are patrilineal or matrilineal and possible implications for gender relations. As the epidemic even in areas with the same farming system manifests itself with marked regional and even local variations, attention needs to be paid to differences between and within regions, districts and communities (see Barnett et al., 1995). A historical perspective can also provide valuable insights: Where available, earlier (anthropological) studies on certain areas or farming systems can be a useful starting point to either understand changes that have taken place over time, possibly due to the epidemic, or to become aware of inherent features of an agricultural system which might have come under strain, do not exist any longer or have been modified. Barnett et al. (1995) mention an example of how such insights can be used: They quote earlier work from the 1950s and early 1960s in Zambia which has shown that matrilineal peoples seem more immediately vulnerable to the effects of labour loss due to the fact that matrilineal households show more instability. Such knowledge can help identify special vulnerability or act as a starting point to understand impact and design interventions.

The following will give an overview over the most important studies carried out on HIV/AIDS and agriculture that can be accessed in and from the Netherlands, starting with impact on farming systems, followed by impact on rural livelihoods, and finally impact at household level, by far the most common type of studies available to date. Some of these studies overlap this categorisation, and their findings will be presented where relevant. Additionally, two sectors which to date have not attracted much research will be briefly discussed: the estate sector and pastoralism. Then a summary of the most important insights from these studies is given, followed by a brief conclusion.

2. HIV/AIDS impact on agricultural production systems

One of the earliest studies on the potential impact of HIV/AIDS on farming systems, the desk study by Gillespie (1989) on Rwanda, already anticipated much of what was to be confirmed by later field-based studies. Gillespie identifies as the crucial issue the labour economy of households, what has in later studies been identified as the interface between domestic and farm labour demand, and its spatial and temporal dimensions (Barnett et al., 1995).

Gillespie's study predicts that the short-term household-level impact of an AIDS death leads to the reallocation of remaining household labour. Longer term impact then leads to a possible change in household composition or the dissolution of households, with the possible consequence of a long-term effect on the agricultural system, visible for example in a change in cropping patterns.

The study divides Rwanda into five different farming systems, differentiated by altitude, soil, and population density (based on a major World Bank study). It then categorises these rural production systems in terms of their sensitivity to AIDS related labour loss. Looking even further, on the regional level a possible loss of human control over ecological systems is predicted: Soil fertility, having in the past been maintained by labour intensive methods, might decline, bushland might return and with it Tsetse fly populations, the incidence of sleeping sickness, and increased livestock mortality and human morbidity, all setting off a downward spiral. More than twenty years later, many of these early predictions have come true for high prevalence areas in some parts of sub-Saharan Africa. While Gillespie's work on Rwanda predates the genocide, since which the parameters of Rwandan farming systems have changed, his methodology used in the classification of farming systems is still a useful tool to understand the impact of HIV/AIDS on such systems, as it can be applied to different contexts.

Such studies, however, need to be complemented by empirical data on how households and communities do actually cope with the circumstances created by the epidemic. Looking at farming systems only is an approach too narrow in that it does not take into account the diversity of livelihoods that farmers exhibit and the potential they have to diversify into activities that are less labour dependent (Haddad & Gillespie, 2001a). The resourcefulness of rural households might be underestimated, leading to inaccurate predictions of the impact at farming system level.

Barnett & Blaikie (1992) in their study on Uganda combine household level impact studies based on extensive fieldwork with farming system classification. Ugandan farming systems are analysed according to their patterns of labour use, including seasonal peaks demanded by certain crops currently grown, crops these could be substituted for without ecological constraints, and typical arrangements for organising labour within the household according to gender and age. Based upon these considerations, an algorithm for Farming System Vulnerability Mapping (FSVM) is developed, classifying and ranking farming systems in Uganda according to their potential vulnerability to labour loss as a result of AIDS.

Subsequent studies covering the impact of the epidemic on farming systems and based on field data include a study carried out by multidisciplinary teams in Uganda, Tanzania and Zambia in 1994 (Barnett et al., 1995), and partly the study by Mongi (2002) in Kenya, and Rugalema (1999) in Tanzania. Both of the latter focus on a particular farming system and how HIV/AIDS impact at household level over time alters that system.

Taken together, studies of HIV/AIDS impact on farming systems can provide the basis for a broad vulnerability mapping of countries: In a first step, different farming systems within a country or region are mapped based on available data. These maps can be overlaid onto sentinel surveillance data to provide an initial guide to the relative vulnerability of different farming systems, from where in due course more detailed analyses and policy responses can be developed (see Barnett et al., 1995).

While such a classification can be a very useful tool indeed, it has been argued that the categorisation of farming systems solely by their degree of vulnerability to AIDS-induced labour loss might be too narrow. Rugalema (1999) argues for example that if the algorithm developed by Barnett & Blaikie (1992) was applied to the Tanzanian farming systems which were at the centre of his study, these would have been classified as very resilient. On the ground, however, his study found that the majority of households afflicted or affected by HIV/AIDS was in fact impoverished, and changes in the farming system occurred as a consequence. Based on these findings the study argues that other assets might be as central to household production and reproduction, and that the loss of labour not withstanding, the degree to which households dispose of their assets relative to their asset base can be an equally important indicator of vulnerability of subsistence farming and livelihood and farming systems to HIV/AIDS (Rugalema, 1999).

Based on these reasonings, the need to go beyond FSVM has been stated, and a Livelihood Vulnerability Mapping (LVM) been suggested (Topouzis, 2000). LVM would include non-agronomic indicators to measure such things as asset depletion; loss of agricultural knowledge and skills; orphaning rates; changes in (women's) time allocation; changes in children's school attendance and nutrition, to name jut the most important. Both, FSVM and LVM could be linked to existing agricultural information and early warning systems. The notion of vulnerability of specific rural production systems to labour loss as presented in FSVM could be linked to the United Nations Food and Agricultural Organisation's (FAO) early warning system concerning drought. LVM could be integrated with FAO's Food Insecurity and Vulnerability Mapping System to broaden it to identify vulnerable livelihoods and livelihood options appropriate in the context of HIV/AIDS (IFAD, 2001; Topouzis, 2000).

3. HIV/AIDS impact on rural livelihoods

A good starting point to understand impact at the rural livelihood level or the level of rural society is Topouzis (1998). Rural society is here seen as a living organism, and the systematic impact of the epidemic depicted as a series of attacks on its immune system, which in turn lead to a host of chain reactions as the society and its varies organs try to fight back and adjust. Topouzis points out that the impact of the epidemic has to be seen cross-sectorally, as the epidemic tends to exacerbate existing problems of rural development like poverty, food insecurity and malnutrition through its catalytic effects and systematic impact (Topouzis, 1998). While these impacts can be exemplified in concrete in looking at the household level, analysing HIV/AIDS impact in connection to rural livelihoods facilitates the understanding of the epidemic as not only affecting individual households but livelihood options. These options can be affected positively or negatively: Beuman (2001) in her study in Uganda for example investigates changes in community dynamics and shows how social ties are weakening, in the process closing off certain livelihood choices. In contrast, as a consequence of the epidemic inter household co-operation might be strengthened and livelihood choices expanded in due course, as has for example been reported from southern Uganda, where self-help groups have been formed in an area where such co-operation used not to be the norm (Barnett & Haslwimmer, 1995; see also NAADS, 2003)

To understand the dynamics between HIV/AIDS and rural livelihoods more broadly, Haddad and Gillespie look at HIV/AIDS impact in the context of the livelihoods framework: In analysing the impact of the epidemic on human, financial, social, physical and natural capital, they show how HIV/AIDS strips individuals, households, networks and communities of assets in these five categories (Haddad & Gillespie, 2001a; 2001b; see also Seeley, 2003; Stokes, 2003). Comparative case study research has shown that livelihood groups' different responses to additional cost in the face of HIV/AIDS related illness or death is indeed determined by their asset base and respective livelihood strategies, and the more diversified the latter, the more options are available.

It has to be pointed out, however, that some of these response strategies might be leading to destitution: Haddad & Gillespie (2001a; 2001b) observed strategies in which tomorrow's livelihoods are being sacrificed in order to hang on to today's, as for example children are pulled out of school to bolster a family's ability to provide care or maintain its current livelihood activities. These findings point to the need to eventually look beyond the level of livelihood analysis and include the wider national system (and in a further step the global political economy, but the latter is beyond the overview given in this piece). This last point shall be exemplified using the example of Uganda: There a switch from cash crops into food crops has been reported among afflicted households, together with a reluctance of farmers to adopt recommended agronomic practices to achieve higher yields (NAADS, 2003). While this change in livelihood strategies might on the face of it be a viable strategy for individual households, it has wider implications for the national economy as the modernisation of agriculture towards cash crops is the most important national policy regarding agricultural production and securing the food requirements of the nation (NAADS, 2003).

More generally it has been argued that what is needed are strategies to enhance the resilience of livelihood systems to any shock, which is implied will at the same time reduce susceptibility and vulnerability of households to the HIV/AIDS epidemic (Chopra, 2003). A similar approach is advocated by Devereux (2003), who - taking the example of the food crisis of southern Africa in 2002 which is described as related to the HIV/AIDS epidemic - argues that this crisis should not be analysed as an emergency at household level, but as a livelihood crisis at community level which requires an integrated approach that addresses the underlying causes of vulnerability. Inspite of an emerging consensus that HIV/AIDS affects all aspects of rural livelihoods and that effective analysis requires a contextual understanding unique to a given geographical area and kinship group, the focus of analysis when looking at HIV/AIDS impact remains often limited to the household level.

4. HIV/AIDS impact at rural household level

Almost all research to date has identified as the most immediate impact of HIV/AIDS at household level its effect on the human capital base in terms of the availability and allocation of labour (White & Robinson, 2000), followed or accompanied by a loss of (financial) assets. While some of the effects of HIV/AIDS mirror those in the wake of shocks like droughts or floods, it has been suggested that others are specific to the particular dynamics through which AIDS configures with household characteristics. Here of special importance is the way in which AIDS undermines and removes labour resources of young adults in the prime of their productive years (Baylies, 2002).

Within the context of rural households, through the loss of labour, often coupled with the loss of urban remittances, it has been shown that HIV/AIDS can have a direct impact on agricultural production in terms of a reduction in cultivated land; a decline in crop yields and the variety of crops cultivated; and changes in livestock (Barnett & Blaikie, 1992; Panos Institute, 1992; for a discussion of livestock in particular see Engh et al., 2000). A still widely quoted graphic example of what might happen once HIV/AIDS enters a household is the idealized longitudinal model Barnett & Blaikie (1992) developed based on their research in Rakai district in Uganda, which shows the different stages of a household's experience of the AIDS epidemic and incorporates all the aspects mentioned above.

The dynamics which unfold within AIDS afflicted rural households pose a threat to the food security of such households or worsen an already food insecure situation. The main impact of the epidemic on rural households practicing smallholder agriculture can thus be analysed as related to the food security status of such households and the individuals belonging to it, as food security is a basic need without which survival itself is put into question and being food insecure is the most critical indicator of a household's vulnerability. It has been shown that HIV/AIDS has affected and predicted that it will continue to affect the ability of households to access food in the quantities and quality necessary for household members to lead an active and healthy life. In those parts of Africa where the epidemic has matured, households are facing labour shortages, downshifting in cropping systems and livestock management, a declining asset base, often exorbitant health care costs, and a breakdown of social solidarity and social bonds - all of which contribute to food insecurity (Barnett, 2003). A study carried out in a village in the Kagera district of Tanzania for example reports a reduction in food consumption by most AIDS afflicted households, while more generally food security is considered to be in jeopardy because, related to the impact of the epidemic, women are no longer able to produce the same amounts of supplementary root cops (Tibaijuka, 1997). Research in West Africa has shown that the most immediate problem for many AIDS-afflicted female headed households is not medical treatment and drugs, but food and malnutrition (Black-Michaud, 1997).

In looking at HIV/AIDS impact in terms of food security at household level, one needs however to take into account that many rural households today have a rather diversified portfolio of livelihood activities, thus the loss of labour might not in every case be the single most important impact (Ellis, 2003).[4] Some studies indicate that a shortage of resources overshadows labour shortages as a constraint encountered by HIV/AIDS afflicted households, leaving households for example unable to purchase necessary agricultural inputs (see for example Kwaramba, 1998). In a similar vein, Rugalema (1999), based on findings from his research in Tanzania, argues that for many widow-headed households in one particular village the main problem after the death of their spouse is cash income rather than labour shortage. A similar point is argued by Tibaijuka (1997) in her Tanzanian study: She found the cost of hired labour to have increased tremendously due to high mortality rates among migrant farm workers. Thus, women-

---

[4] Ellis (2003) argues - based on broader livelihood research - that all rural households straddle farm and non-farm activities. The most successful construct non-farm components into their livelihood portfolio that comprise activities not related to agriculture. The least successful remain in subsistence agriculture and undertake low-wage casual labour on other farms. He suggests that the key to rising farm productivity and by implication better food security are urban and non-farm economic growth, not farm output on its own.

headed households dependent on migrant labour could not afford wage cost any longer, had to carry out the tasks usually carried out by hired labour themselves, and experienced a drop in production as a consequence.

Research carried out by the Food Economy Group (2002a, 2002b) in Makueni district, Kenya, shows how households at the top end of the wealth breakdown are the key to food security of those at the bottom end, as they will hire a considerable amount of farm labour. Resources to secure food for poor households at the research site came to 50 percent from agricultural labour for wealthier households. HIV/AIDS has so far mainly hit these richer households, who in turn have incurred higher expenditure on health, while at the same time decreasing the amount of money spent on hiring labour - a move which threatens the food security of poorer households. It is asserted that when one of the richer households is afflicted with HIV/AIDS, this is likely to have a direct impact on the income of and food availability within three or more poorer households (Food Economy Group 2002a).[5]

Studies like these indicate two things: Firstly, the main focus on labour might need to be reconsidered when looking at HIV/AIDS impact on rural smallholders. Additionally, in an environment in which agricultural production systems revert back to more subsistence farming in the face of the epidemic, the question arises how the landless or those with little land who depend on rural employment for their survival will do so, whether themselves directly afflicted or affected by the epidemic or not.

Secondly, it has been suggested that it might be necessary to move beyond the current emphasis on individual households as unit of analysis in order to factor the complex linkages and networks between households and extended families and communities (Topouzis, 2000). As an alternative concept the 'cluster' as a social unit has been suggested: A 'cluster' is defined by Drinkwater (1994) as a group of producers between whom multiple resource exchanges, usually based

---

[5] Food security in general can be realised (following Sen) through 'exchange entitlement' (income earned from on- and off-farm activities) or 'production entitlement' (direct food production).

on kinship, labour, food exchange and possibly common access to draught power are taking place.[6] The concept of 'cluster' might thus allow for a better understanding of relationships between individuals of different generations, gender, marital status, kinship status and so forth, as it allows to understand individuals as themselves, as parts of larger social aggregates, and as parts of representative groups, thus bringing agency and structure into view simultaneously (Drinkwater, 1994). This is of particular importance in looking at the impact of HIV/AIDS, as this impact is experienced twofold, in terms of the deterioration of household economies, as well as in the unravelling of the social fabric of the lives of those afflicted or affected by AIDS (Drinkwater, 2003). Cluster based analysis in a rural area in the south-eastern Midlands of Zimbabwe has for example shown the importance of the impact of illness and death among urban residents on rural households. Urban remittances funded items such as agricultural inputs and school fees, and were overall critical for the maintenance of production and consumption levels across an extended family (Westley cited in Drinkwater, 2003). In addition, findings from Malawi suggest a high frequency of changes in marriage partners (possibly connected to HIV/AIDS, though this hypothesis has not been further investigated) and thus show the fluid and fragile identity of the household itself (Shah et al., 2003). Cluster analysis might also help to pick up lost threads from dissolved households (see for example Mutangadura, 2000, who reports that 65 percent of households featuring in her study ceased to exist) as well as trace surviving orphans. Finally, cluster analysis can demonstrate clearly how the illness or death of one key producer leads to the deterioration of the livelihoods of four or five households, as reported by Drinkwater (2003) in relation to Zambia and Zimbabwe, leading him to argue that if only 20 percent of households in an area are afflicted, this can have a major impact on the locality as a whole and beyond. So far, the 'cluster' has only been used in very few studies dealing with the impact of HIV/AIDS on rural agriculture, thus it is too early to judge how useful and practical it really proves to be.

---

[6] These resources do not entail exchanges based on reciprocity between households and individuals not of the same cluster (Drinkwater, 2003), exchanges which may form the basis of social capital within the wider community.

Generally speaking, the vast majority of impact studies at household level are qualitative studies, done at the micro-level to investigate the effects of HIV/AIDS on rural households and drawn from specific geographic sites purposively chosen because they were known to have high infection rates such as Rakai district in Uganda and Kagera district in Tanzania (see for example Barnett & Blaikie, 1992; Menon et al., 1998; World Bank, 1997). While these studies provide valuable insights into how afflicted and affected households respond to the disease, they are limited in their ability to understand wider levels of impact on the agricultural sector. An attempt to partly fill that gap and quantitatively estimate the effects of the disease on farm production and farm income on a national scale is the study by Yamano & Jayne (2004), based on survey data from Kenya and using economic modelling. Interestingly, their results confirm many of the findings of these smaller scale, qualitative studies they set out to complement.

Many studies dealing with HIV/AIDS impact at household level do not deal explicitly with impact on agriculture in general or food security in particular, but with general economic impact on a household often measured as the loss of assets (see for example Béchu, 1998; Menon et al., 1998). Such studies are, however, a useful supplement to the studies dealing exclusively with agriculture. Quite a number of these studies were conducted among rural communities, where a general economic decline is bound to affect agricultural production and food security, particularly in the face of the fact that few households rely on subsistence agriculture alone these days. Other studies include special sections on agricultural impact, like the study by Armstrong (1995), with sections on smallholder households as well as the farming systems in Uganda.

In general, the overall economic impact of adult death on the surviving household members in rural and urban communities alike varies according to the following sets of characteristics: characteristics of the diseased individual in terms of age, gender, income, and whether the person died of HIV/AIDS or some other cause; characteristics of the household, such as its composition, asset base and relative economic status; characteristics of the community, such as attitudes towards helping needy households and overall availability of resources, as well as social norms, particularly those concerning marriage and inheritance rights; and the timing of sickness or deaths within the household, the duration of sickness, and whether one or more household members fall ill (Shah et al., 2003; World Bank, 1997). These characteristics influence how and if afflicted households can cope.

5. HIV/AIDS impact on the agricultural estate sector

In addition to smallholder agriculture, in some countries in particular it is important to look at the impact of the AIDS epidemic on the estate sector. Taking the example of Kenya, large scale agro estates account for 30 percent of total formal wage labour in the private sector (Rugalema et al., 1999), they thus form an important part of the national economy. To date, the impact of HIV/AIDS on the commercial agricultural sector is less well understood than its impact on the semi-subsistence sector. This is the case inspite of the fact that, being largely dependent on migrant labour, the commercial sector is highly vulnerable to HIV/AIDS, as labourers often live on the estate, away from their families. They can become an important vector for spreading the disease, in particular as social networks tend to be weaker in such settings.

Generalised projections by the FAO predict a loss of around 20 percent in the agricultural labour force through AIDS in the hardest-hit African countries (www.fao.org/hivaids). As a consequence, commercial agriculture is bound to feel the loss of specialised agricultural labour.

The few detailed studies available on the commercial sector, studies which explore the susceptibility and vulnerability of the estate sector and its workers, include the study by Haslwimmer on the Nakambala Sugar Estate in Zambia (in Barnett & Haslwimmer, 1995); the study by Rugalema et al. (1999) on the commercial agricultural sector of Kenya, covering five agro-estates in three different provinces; and most recently the study by Fox et al. (2004) conducted on a tea producing estate in western Kenya and describing the 'natural history' of productivity decline associated with AIDS.

All these studies show the following: Due to HIV related illness agro-estates face rising cost and losses in profits due to loss of workers and working hours. Medical and funeral expenses exceed budget provisions, and terminal benefits (where available to workers), retraining and replacement measures add further to the expenses incurred by the epidemic. All these factors taken together lower the productivity of the enterprise. In addition, Rugalema et al. (1999) report that in individual discussions with workers it was revealed that there are significant psychological effects which are neither easy to measure nor easy to detect: Workers pointed out that they were psychologically unsettled by the frequent illness and death of family members and/or colleagues, all bound to bear on working morale and productivity.

Certain types of labour intensive companies, such as sugar estates, which often heavily depend on out-growers (individual farmers who supply cane to the estate) are particularly hard hit, as cultivation patterns of some afflicted out-growers change to the less labour intensive agricultural production of cassava and maize (Rugalema et al., 1999). This points to the fact that it is often not enough to look at one agricultural sector on its own, as there are many linkages between commercial agriculture and smallholders: The latter might produce for larger estates; often families split with one (or more) members earning cash in the commercial sector, while other members work on the family farm, either for the estate, as subsistence smallholders, or a combination of both. Even where more or all family members can find employment on the same agricultural estate, it is often the case that some members stay behind on the family farm, not least to secure their entitlement to the family land which might be forfeited if it lies shallow.

At the same time, all surveyed estates have social, economic and environmental factors which favour the spread of the epidemic, including poor housing, overcrowding, lack of recreational facilities, and unequal income earning opportunities for men and women. The latter drives women to sell sex to make ends meet (Rugalema et al., 1999). More generally, again using the example of Kenya, agricultural workers are the lowest paid workers in the whole of the Kenyan economy. For men and women alike this makes it often difficult to save enough money for family needs, thus partners or other family members might feel the need to engage in selling sexual favours. In addition, the structure of the workforce lets commercial sex strive to satisfy the needs of both, men and women. While in proportional terms, the study by Rugalema et al. (1999) shows more men were afflicted by the epidemic than women, on one estate it were members of the female workforce which were the major victims of AIDS: That estate was a floriculture company, and horticulture and floriculture companies employ more women than men, as women are regarded as more competent or rather more careful in dealing with tender plants. On such estates, young men survive on providing sex to the female workforce. These so-called 'flower mummies' entice them by providing food and accommodation in return for sex.

More research needs to be done on the impact of the epidemic on the commercial sector and its linkages with smallholder agriculture and other parts of the nationwide economy. To end, it should be pointed out that, if managed properly, the commercial agricultural sector can also be a force for good in fighting the epidemic in the sense that it can provide information and training on prevention as well as health care facilities. In addition, the sector might offer opportunities for AIDS orphans to learn some essential agricultural skills (Haddad & Gillespie, 2001a).

6. HIV/AIDS impact on pastoralism

Despite the fact that pastoralists[7] represent a significant proportion of the rural population in many high HIV prevalence countries where the impact of the epidemic on rural livelihoods has long been felt (examples include Kenya and Uganda), virtually no research has been carried out on how the epidemic might affect pastoralists' livelihoods and production systems (a partial exception is the study by NAADS, 2003, in Uganda; for a discussion of more general studies of such livelihoods see Morton, 2003). Virtually all pastoralist communities are heavily vulnerable to external shocks such as droughts, often coupled with armed conflict and encroachment on rangelands, a fact which might render them highly susceptible to HIV infection, if findings from the wider literature on HIV/AIDS and agricultural livelihoods are anything to go by. In addition, spatial mobility has been defined as the crucial factor determining the pathways of the spread of the epidemic in western Africa, thus pastoralists whose livelihood depends on migratory patterns should be a central focus of concern in that region (Black-Michaud, 1997). As no data is available to date on sero-prevalence disaggregated to include pastoralists as a category, the state of the epidemic among pastoralist communities is simply not known.

Morton (2003) identifies a number of other characteristics potentially making pastoralists particularly susceptible and vulnerable to HIV/AIDS. These include sexual networking traditions among certain pastoralist societies in eastern Africa; mobility patterns; and exclusion from health education and services, often even among pastoralists who moved to towns as labour migrants. What has been said about HIV/AIDS impact in relation to agricultural communities in general also applies to pastoralists: certain characteristics of their livelihood system might make them highly susceptible and vulnerable to the epidemic, while other characteristics might contribute to resilience and resistance. Research is urgently needed to investigate these dynamics among different pastoralist communities, not only in eastern Africa but equally in the neighbouring countries to the North (including

---

[7] A pastoralist production system is defined as one in which 50 percent or more of gross household revenue comes from livestock or livestock-related activities (see Morton, 2003).

Somalia, Sudan, Ethiopia and Eritrea), in some of which the effects of HIV/AIDS have not been felt so strongly (yet) but with whom a variety of cross-border linkages exist, and also beyond the region (for example in Namibia, Botswana, the Sahel and North Africa).

7. The impact of HIV/AIDS on rural livelihoods - the evidence so far

It can not be repeated often enough: Most of what has been presented so far as 'knowledge' about the impact of HIV/AIDS on rural households and agriculture has been based on a limited number of studies, usually carried out in small areas, often single villages, in eastern and southern Africa, to date the epicentre of the epidemic.[8] Given the spatial and temporal specificities of the epidemic, generalisations from such micro-studies can be misleading, and their findings become problematic when treated as a more generalised truth, in particular with regard to the fact that within each country HIV/AIDS has its own origin, geographic pattern of dispersion, and affects particular population groups in different ways (White & Robinson, 2000). In spite of this dearth of data, statements referring to the actual or potential impact of the epidemic on rural livelihoods are routinely made and cited repeatedly thereafter, in most cases without (sufficient) empirical evidence (Topouzis, 2000). This is particular the case concerning such hard to measure impacts as the lessening of social ties or the loss of socially reproductive labour. Having said that, however, if treated with sufficient caution, small scale research carried out among particular communities can provide useful material to inform the situation elsewhere.

A brief summary of what has been observed as the impact of HIV/AIDS on agricultural production and food security within rural households in different settings in sub-Saharan Africa includes the following points: loss of (young) adult on and off farm labour leading to a decline in production; decline in income, leading to decreased food

---

[8] A forthcoming study carried out in Benue state in Nigeria does, however, indicate that some of the coping strategies observed in eastern and southern Africa can be observed in parts of western Africa as well. At the same time, the case is made for country-specific analysis and caution is urged in assuming that scenarios develop similarly (van Liere, M., T. Hilhorst & C. de Koning, draft title 'The impact of HIV/AIDS in Benue: Implications for rural livelihoods', Royal Tropical Institute Amsterdam/UK Department for International Development, forthcoming; email exchange with Thea Hilhorst, 02 July 2004). See also the FAO study on western Africa by Black-Michaud (1997).

consumption, increased drop-out among schoolchildren, and poorer health and nutrition status; erosion of the household asset base through depletion of savings and forced disposal of productive assets; rise in expenditure for medical treatment, transport and funeral costs; demographic changes, most prominently an increase in the household dependency ratio with a higher number of dependents relying on smaller numbers of productive household members; loss of agricultural knowledge, practices and skills (for example farm and livestock management and marketing skills); loss of social capital as kinship networks are overstretched and with it a disruption of social security mechanisms and changes in inter-household relationships; altered values within the community - young farmers for example have been observed not to be interested in farming any longer as even early maturing crops are regarded as a long term investment and one might die before reaping the benefits; potentially less well-managed communal resources; depression and lack of motivation as a consequence of the psychological impact of illness and death (see Barnett & Haslwimmer, 1995; IFAD, 2001; de Waal & Tumushabe, 2003 for a more detailed discussion).

At sectoral level, concerning the African rural sector HIV/AIDS induced morbidity and mortality result among other things in the decimation of skilled as well as unskilled agricultural labour, combined with changes in the age structure and quality of the agricultural labour force as more elderly people and children assume greater roles in farming - and as a consequence a decline in overall agricultural output on smallholder as well as commercial farms; capacity erosion and disruption in service delivery of formal and informal rural institutions (for a discussion of HIV/AIDS impact on agricultural extension services see Bota et al., 2001; Qamar, 2001; Topouzis, 2003); decline in public health status, including increased malnutrition as a consequence of loss of income and assets; wider social impacts including a drop in educational level as children are taken out of school, the marginalisation of youth, and an increase in the number of child or orphan headed and/or grandparents headed households (White & Robinson, 2000).

On a broader scale, a generalised HIV/AIDS epidemic in combination with other shocks like droughts or floods might create what has been termed a 'new variant famine', a new kind of acute food crisis in which there is no expectation of a return to either sustainable livelihoods or a demographic equilibrium (de Waal & Tumushabe, 2003; de Waal & Whiteside, 2003).

8. Gender as the decisive factor

One issue that emerges from this summary is the importance of gender attributes to adequately understand and eventually address the impact of HIV/AIDS on agricultural production systems in general and household food security in particular. The main impact of HIV/AIDS induced morbidity and mortality can be described as the disruption of the household productive-domestic labour interface, which in rural agricultural economies primarily affects women. Smallholder farming in particular is characterised by a close relationship between household domestic activities (childcare, food processing, home maintenance) and production activities. Women are at the centre of this interface as food producers, custodians of food security, and caregivers (Topouzis, 1999). Female morbidity and mortality can thus be assumed to have a particularly dramatic impact on a household's well-being in general and household food security in particular, while male adult morbidity and mortality might leave the surviving widow in a precarious situation.

A number of studies which show the gender dimension of HIV/AIDS impact on rural households - often without specifically setting out to investigate it, but as one of their findings - support these assumptions. The most important findings from some of these studies are the following:

Gillespie (1989) predicts that a female AIDS death would reduce nuclear household agricultural labour input by over 50 percent, as many agricultural tasks - in particular those concerning food crops - are traditionally women's tasks. These predictions lead him to propagate an increasing need for the development of appropriate technology for reducing drudgery in unpaid women's work, not only in agriculture, but equally and perhaps more crucially concerning the domestic sphere as well - the importance of the latter is equally stressed by Barnett & Blaikie (1992). Barnett & Haslwimmer (1995) report for all three countries in their study - Zambia, Uganda and Tanzania - that the loss of male household members has a significant impact on the management of the household economy and the marketing of agricultural produce, as many female-headed households have to rely on middle men who often exploit them. On the other hand, data from Malawi illustrates that households that experienced a recent active male adult death have 32 percent less area planted than households that have experienced a recent female death - this is due to the fact that land preparation is heavy work usually carried out by men (SADC FANR, 2003).

The findings reported above demonstrate that the local gender division of labour together with other gender disparities are bound to determine the manner and severity of the impact of HIV/AIDS on rural households. At the same time, the epidemic is bound to have an impact on the dynamics of gender relations.

Some studies have shown that the epidemic worsens gender disparities. Taking the example of Malawi, evidence exists that in the event of the husband's death, surviving widows are being pushed into economic and social destitution, due to the likelihood of the widow to lose property or to fail to manage the farm enterprise. Similar findings are reported from Namibia and Uganda. For certain areas of Namibia, Engh et al. (2000) show that upon death of their spouse widows lose most or even all of the livestock on which their livelihood is based. From Uganda, Topouzis with Hemrich (1994) report that - partly due to the stigma attached to surviving women when it is suspected their husbands have died of AIDS - widows are being left ostracized and deprived of the traditional social security mechanisms for widows to fall back on. On the other hand, a study conducted among rural households in Siaya district in Kenya by Opiyo (2001) found that widows often adapt better and develop more sustainable coping strategies than widowers.

A study that specifically set out to investigate a possible change in traditional gender roles in connection with the HIV/AIDS epidemic is the study by Waller (1997) in Zambia. Women's crops in the study area have always been essential for the household's food security. Even before the onset of HIV/AIDS due to other shocks in the area many households were already vulnerable and food insecure, a fact which made them more dependent on women's agricultural activities, including growing food crops and market gardening. With HIV/AIDS induced morbidity, the burden of care falls disproportionally on women. Their incomes are thus being drawn into conflicting expenditures between farming inputs and care giving. Indeed, women's cash returns from market gardening are being invested in care rather than farming. At the same time, the amount of women's time that goes into caring is not available for weeding and planting, tasks men do not take over as traditionally these are women's tasks. Overall, women spend less time in their fields, productivity and food security decline, starting of an often downward spiral from which the household might not recover and dissolve (Waller, 1997). Waller's study shows how a failure to change traditional gender roles makes adaptation to the additional threat posed by HIV/AIDS almost impossible.

In this context it needs to be pointed out that also positive changes in gender dynamics have been reported. From Uganda, there is for example evidence that parents start to leave a will behind making their daughters an eligible heir, something never seen before. In addition, some widows begin to own important productive resources and household assets through inheritance, where traditionally they were only allowed to keep property related to their reproductive activities. In families were a woman falls ill, male members have started to spend time with cooking or fetching firewood, traditionally female tasks (NAADS, 2003). In general the HIV/AIDS epidemic can become the starting point for dynamic processes leading to more flexible gender roles and possibly more gender equality in the longer term.

Many of the studies discussed above, it has to be pointed out, reflect a specific epidemiological stage of the epidemic: A stage where the majority of death where male household heads, and the problems of widows left behind became severe. Meanwhile, the pattern of the epidemic has changed and more women become infected and at an increasingly younger age than men. Young adult female morbidity and mortality is thus likely to alter the impact on rural households and smallholder agriculture in the future - and may render surviving widowers or other single male headed households particularly vulnerable.

Altogether, the impact of the pandemic on rural agricultural systems and gender relations has to be seen as a dynamic and systematic process, not a linear sequence (Topouzis, 2000). For the time being, a general tendency of the impact of the epidemic seems the fact that young adult male labour loss has more serious consequences for agricultural intensification and the macro-parameters of agricultural production, whereas young female adult labour loss is more closely related to household food security, malnutrition, child withdrawal from school[9] and the appearance of orphan headed households (Topouzis, 2000; for the latter claims see also Mutangadura, 2000).

Taken together, the HIV/AIDS epidemic brings to the fore decades of failure in development policies to give women more control over their lives. It has been suggested that low income, income inequality and low status of women are all highly associated with high levels of HIV infection (Drimie, 2002a, citing World Bank research). Inequities in gender roles run parallel to inequities in income and assets, including the essential asset for rural households, access to land. Such inequalities are often a result of unequal power relations within rural households, and can leave women particularly vulnerable to the impact of the epidemic as well as susceptible to infection.[10]

The epidemic thus exacerbates already present social, economic and cultural inequalities between genders, and mitigation strategies need to tackle these issues to be long term sustainable.

An important gap in present knowledge is the systematic impact of the epidemic on gender roles in agricultural production (apart from such individual studies as cited above). While it is generally argued

---

[9] Concerning the withdrawal of children from school, it is commonly assumed that girls are withdrawn more quickly and in higher numbers. But this 'knowledge' has to be taken with a pinch of salt: The study by Waller (1997) in Zambia shows that specifically in southern Province teenage boys are more vulnerable to be taken out of school since the livelihood there depends largely on cattle herding, an activity carried out by boys. This once more points to the importance of looking at particular farming practices and gender dimensions within these, and be weary of rough and ready generalisations.

[10] It has to be noted here that power relations are different from community to community and in general are a dynamic process - a very good study of such relations is the collection by Waterhouse and Vijfhuizen (2001) in different rural contexts of Mozambique.

that small differences in terms of more equitable gender roles among households and communities can have a positive impact on food security in households afflicted or affected by the epidemic, and that the more food secure households are those in which both genders are involved in diverse agricultural production practices (Topouzis, 1999), little is known about the gender context of households that are able to cope with the impact of HIV/AIDS and recover from food insecurity.

9. HIV/AIDS and other livelihood shocks

Apart from this lack of knowledge on gender dynamics, a central question remains: Is HIV/AIDS different from other disasters? Rugalema (2000) argues that coping in the face of AIDS is derived from famine literature which might be ill suited to analyse household responses to HIV/AIDS. In contrast, White & Robinson (2000) argue that lessons might be learned from other shocks on how to cope with HIV/AIDS. They criticise that much of the household level research on the impact of HIV/AIDS has not drawn on the substantial existing literature on shocks to rural households and the responding coping strategies they adopt (White & Robinson, 2000). One of the few studies relating AIDS to other shocks is Waller (1997): While she acknowledges the general difficulty of disentangling the impact of HIV/AIDS from that of other shocks, her study shows how traditional responses to such shocks have been undercut for HIV/AIDS afflicted and/or affected households due to labour shortages coupled with medical or transport expenses. She argues that HIV/AIDS compounded with other shocks has generally reduced household food security and overall economic productivity (see also Baylies, 2003, on a discussion of different shocks). Similarly, Kwaramba (1998) compares households were AIDS deaths have occurred with those where other deaths have occurred and comes to the conclusion that while both types of households experience a decline in agricultural output, this decline is more drastic within AIDS afflicted households, while at the same time other coping mechanisms might be compromised.

In general, however, it has been observed that most of the research that examines the socio-economic impact of HIV/AIDS has rarely drawn upon previous models developed in the context of the impact of different shocks on rural households, their coping mechanisms, and household vulnerability. A clear theoretical framework is thus lacking which places HIV/AIDS firmly within the context of these other processes - and here the AWLAE programme could help to fill a gap in theory, in particular the research carried out by Lydia Ndirangu in Kenya.[11]

Rather than investigating impact and mitigation strategies as stemming from a root cause - HIV/AIDS as a single factor causing poverty and vulnerability - these issues can perhaps more usefully be understood in relation to the resources available to households and the nature of the enabling or disenabling environment, which are the key factors that define available livelihood strategies and affect a household's resilience to shock and its vulnerability (White & Robinson, 2000). Within such a more holistic approach, the gender division of labour and the social networks available to women as different from men might be crucial, and a more systematic knowledge of these parameters, not only in response to the impact of HIV/AIDS but equally to other shocks, be they less severe or not, is called for.

---

[11] The working title of Lydia Ndirangu's PhD research is 'Risk Management and Poverty in Rural Kenya'. She examines the effects of different shocks, among them HIV/AIDS, on portfolio choice and the ability of individual household members to keep consumption smooth over time and relative to other members of the household in the middle and lower agro-ecological zones of Thika and Maragwa district in Central Kenya.

10. Some concluding remarks

From what has been said so far, it follows that the impact of HIV/AIDS on agricultural production systems and rural livelihoods can, at the end of the day, not be separated from the macro economy and the wider societal environment. In spite of that fact, studies undertaken on HIV/AIDS and its impact on agriculture tend to be limited to showing the impact of the epidemic on cropping patterns, yields, nutritional status, or specific population, but largely fail to consider issues such as a change in prices of commodities, or land tenure rights of women and children (du Guerny, 2002). The latter has of late partly changed, as the importance of land issues for the severity of HIV/AIDS impact on households and communities in general, and widows, single mothers and surviving children in particular has been recognised (see Drimie, 2002a; 2002b). The AWLAE programme can make an important contribution here in providing more research-based evidence, most prominently the research project carried out by Gaynor Paradza on women's entitlement to land in the times of AIDS in the communal areas of Zimbabwe.[12]

In addition, it is widely acknowledged that urban and rural economies are intrinsically linked, with incomes within the rural environment often depending upon wages earned within the urban environment. For southern Africa for example, smallholder agriculture has been shown to have become impossible without inputs from labour migrant remittances, a fact that underpins the complexity of rural livelihoods (Drimie, 2002a). This implies that the impact of HIV/AIDS on the formal, largely urban based economies will increasingly affect cash flows between the two sectors (Drimie, 2002a) - while at the same time the costs of AIDS are largely borne by rural communities, as infected city dwellers often return to their communities once they fall ill (Topouzis, 1998). Moreover, economic development in itself might contribute to the spread of HIV/AIDS in rural areas by strengthening rural-urban linkages and mobility, as has been shown for example in the case of Botswana (Topouzis, 1998). To understand and be able to mitigate the impact of HIV/AIDS on rural livelihoods it is thus

---

[12] Gaynor Paradza carries out a research project entitled 'HIV/AIDS and Gendered Access to Land in Chikwaka Communal Area of Zimbabwe'.

necessary to have an understanding of both, the role of land and subsistence practices for small-scale agriculture, as well as the broader labour market and macro-economic environment, as the latter underpins incomes within the rural economy and rural households' diverse livelihood strategies.

Eventually, responses to the epidemic need to be associated with central questions of social and economic policy, with questions of poverty, its origins, its endurance and alleviation. As such, the spread of the epidemic within rural populations is linked to these populations' vulnerability, resulting in part from a failure in (rural) development (du Guerny, 2002). Where poverty alleviation in rural communities simply aims to adjust households to the market in shoring up their assets and building the 'capacity' of their members, without addressing deeper inequalities around gender, class, age, disability and so on which systematically obstruct the realisation of capabilities, it has failed in the past and is even more prone to fail in the future in the face of the challenges posed by HIV/AIDS. Only if programmes of poverty alleviation and food security are constructed around and address the factors which drive the epidemic and determine its impact at household level can the epidemic be contained and rural development be achieved (Baylies, 2002).

Responses to the epidemic need to centre on examining what has been called the two-way-linkages between HIV/AIDS and rural livelihoods (Loevinsohn & Gillespie, 2003): How are elements within agricultural livelihoods - livelihoods embedded into the larger national and global political economy - increasing or decreasing the risk of HIV infection, and how are they helping to mitigate or enhance the impact of AIDS.

Part 2 – Annotated bibliography

1. HIV/AIDS and agriculture

Bangwe, L. (1997) *Agricultural Change under Structural Adjustment and Other Shocks in Monze District, Zambia*. Bath: University of Bath. http://www.bath.ac.uk/~hssjgc/lewis1.html.

This study needs to be read together with the study by Waller (1997). It discusses some of the adaptation mechanisms to different shocks, including Structural Adjustment Programmes, drought and cattle disease in Monze district in Zambia, without specifically making reference to the huge amount of time spent in health related activities due to HIV/AIDS (the latter task is carried out by Waller). The question is posed whether (and in what way) these strategies might also be useful in coping with HIV/AIDS, or whether the epidemic might actually compromise these strategies. To distinguish the impact of HIV/AIDS on rural households from other shocks it is proposed to chose a high HIV prevalence study area for which baseline data is available before or at the early stages of the epidemic (baseline data ideally reflecting other periodically occurring shocks), so that both sets of data can be compared.

Barnett, T. (2003) 'HIV/AIDS has changed the world: Food insecurity and disease - what we need to know', *The Courier ACP-EU* **197**, pp. 50-51.

Barnett, T., J. **Tumushabe**, G. **Bantebya**, R. **Ssebuliba**, J. **Ngasongwa**, D. **Kapinga**, M. **Ndelike**, M. **Drinkwater**, G. **Mitti** and M. **Haslwimmer** (1995) 'The Social and Economic Impact of HIV/AIDS on Farming Systems and Livelihoods in Rural Africa: Some Experience and Lessons from Uganda, Tanzania and Zambia', *Journal of International Development* **7**, pp. 163-176.

This article, based on research undertaken in Uganda, Tanzania and Zambia in the late 1980s and early 1990s, describes some of the effects of HIV/AIDS on rural communities in these countries. It further predicts some of the medium term impacts of the epidemic, while at the same time noting the difficulty to generalise about its effects, as impact varies considerably between and within communities. The key issue in all three studies was found to be the interface between domestic and farm labour demands and the vulnerability of rural livelihood systems to labour loss, spatially as well as temporarily. Policy responses thus need to be formulated on the basis of the known temporal and spatial differentiation of the epidemic and ultimately together with wider social and economic policies (see also Barnett & Haslwimmer, 1995).

Barnett, T. and M. **Haslwimmer** (1995) *Effects of HIV/AIDS on farming systems in Eastern Africa*. Rome: FAO.
http://www.fao.org/docrep/V4710E/V4710E00.htm.

This publication discusses in more detail the issues raised in Barnett et al. (1995) in relation to the impact of the HIV/AIDS epidemic on farming systems in Tanzania, Uganda and Zambia. While the results prove to be quite divers, not only between countries but equally between different agricultural systems in the same country, as the main cost of the epidemic to a society the following issues have been identified: a loss of output, primarily due to the heavy dependence upon labour power (paid and unpaid) in all three countries' farming systems; this is compounded by the less easily estimated social as well as economic cost associated with the burden of looking after orphans, care, and costs associated with the disruption of socialisation and education of the young. One chapter focuses on the agricultural estate sector, discussing in detail the case of the Nakambala Sugar Estate in Zambia among others.

Barnett, T. and P. **Blaikie** (1992) *AIDS in Africa. Its present and future impact*. London: Belhaven Press.

This book is one of the first major studies on the social and economic impact of HIV/AIDS in Africa, based on demographic, sociological and anthropological data from field research carried out in rural Uganda. AIDS is defined as a long wave disaster, thus coping strategies need to pay attention to the gradual onset of its impact. Downstream social and economic effects at household level are described from the perspective of individuals, who are categorised as members of afflicted, affected, or not directly touched (unaffected) households. Furthermore, coping mechanisms that have been developed in the worst affected areas of Rakai district at household, family and community level are presented, and the question of AIDS orphans is discussed. The concept of vulnerability to the epidemic is explored particularly clearly in taking the example of the social and economic risk environment, the 'ecology of risk', in Buganda. Finally, impact on farming systems is dealt with and an algorithm is developed for classifying different farming systems according to their vulnerability to the loss of labour as a result of AIDS.

Baylies, C. (2002) 'The Impact of AIDS on Rural Households in Africa: A Shock Like Any Other?', *Development and Change* **33**, pp. 611-632.

The article starts from the observation that in areas where HIV prevalence is high, household production can be significantly affected and the integrity of households compromised. Yet, policy responses to the impact of the epidemic have been muted, particularly when compared with responses to droughts or other emergencies. Looking at data from Zambia, as one reason for this under-reaction to AIDS its disappearance into the 'privacy' of afflicted households is identified. It is concluded that effective initiatives to curb the epidemic must attend to the specific features of AIDS, incorporating both an assault on the inequalities which drive the epidemic and sensitivity to the staging of AIDS across and within households. A multi-prolonged approach is advocated which addresses not only mitigation or prevention, but at the same time deeper inequalities around gender, class, disability and so on which systematically obstruct the realisation of capabilities and result in marginalisation and disadvantage, and ultimately prevent rehabilitation and development.

Beuman, J. (2001) *The impact of HIV/AIDS on family relations, and women's ability to cope with insecurities. A research on the management of social and economic insecurities of widows, within the context of the HIV/AIDS epidemic, Nyamiyaga, Mbarara District, Uganda*. Wageningen University, Department of Law and Rural Development.

This thesis has as its starting point that social security presupposes not only the availability of material resources (land, money, and crops) but also of social resources (social relationships, rights, laws, status and power) through which material resources can be transformed into social security provisions. Within the study area, increasing socio-economic differentiation has been observed, with few people in the village owing large plots (partly accumulated through distress sales by AIDS afflicted families), while poor people becoming more dependent on renting plots to secure their food security needs. It is questioned whether the poor can develop coping strategies at all in this set-up, as the data seems to indicate that many decisions taken by the poor are not rational or deliberate, but a form of 'distress-coping'. Overall, the study observes that the community spirit has weakened considerably, as people have become more individualistic and money-minded.

Black-Michaud, A. (1997) *Impact du VIH/SIDA sur les systèmes d'exploitations agricoles en Afrique de l'Ouest (in French)*. Rome: FAO. http://www.fao.org/docrep/W6983F/w6983f01.htm.

This report is meant to complement the study on AIDS and agricultural systems in Uganda, Zambia and Tanzania commissioned by the FAO in 1994 (see Barnett & Haslwimmer, 1995; Barnett et al., 1995). Based on qualitative data collected in semi-structured interviews (154 cases altogether) and focus group discussions, it analyses the repercussions of the epidemic for different agricultural systems in Burkina Faso and Côte d'Ivoire, at the time of the report the two west African countries most severely affected. Furthermore, it describes mitigation strategies as developed by afflicted households and individuals, and proposes future intervention strategies. Four different agricultural zones were chosen for the survey, two in each country. The major difference to the eastern African scenario was found to be the much stronger connection between pathways of the spread of HIV/AIDS and spatial mobility of the population, a fact that was true for all agricultural zones and systems, albeit for different reasons. Apart from that and the fact that overall the severity of the epidemic had not reached the same proportions as in eastern Africa, similar impacts could be observed. These include a reduction in manual labour leading to less land being cultivated, changes in the crops cultivated, lower yields, and a potential threat to food security. A comparison between the mitigation strategies in two agricultural zones in Côte d'Ivoire, Korhogo in the north (savannah condition, often poor soils) and Daloa in centre-west (tropical forest, rich soils) provides a good example of how the conditions of the natural environment determine the leeway for households and individuals to adjust to a shock like HIV/AIDS.

Bota, S., M. **McKey**, G. **Malindi** and P. **Alleyne** (2001) *The Impact of HIV/AIDS on Agricultural Extension Organisation and Field Operations in Selected Countries of sub-Saharan Africa, With Appropriate Institutional Response*. Malawi: FAO and UNDP.

This report presents the findings of a study conducted in Malawi between January 2001 and July 2001 covering various public, parastal, NGO and private organisations and institutions within the agricultural sector. Quantitative as well as qualitative methods of data collection were used, specifically focus group discussions with farmers and extension staff, and structured questionnaire surveys for frontline, supervisory and management staff. The study documents the impact of the epidemic on farming communities in Malawi at household and farming system level, as well as on agricultural extension services. It shows farmers as well as extension workers being aware of the epidemic and willing to talk about it. This awareness, however, has not translated into attitude and behaviour change; in contrast, farmers as well as extension workers are often involved in behaviours and practices likely to put them at risk of HIV infection.

Chopra, M. (2003) *Equity Issues in HIV/AIDS, Nutrition and Food Security in Southern Africa*. Regional Network for Equity in Health in Southern Africa (EQUINET).
http://www.equinetafrica.org/bibl/docs/hivfood.pdf.

The paper starts from the observation that common public health and agricultural services have not significantly reduced the vulnerability or susceptibility of rural people to HIV/AIDS, nor to food insecurity or malnutrition. HIV/AIDS, nutrition and food security are described as interacting at biological, individual, community and national levels, all four of which are linked and reinforce each other. It is suggested that greater awareness of the synergies between nutrition, food security and HIV/AIDS could lead to an approach in which prevention, treatment, rehabilitation and mitigation strategies are combined in ways that reduce vulnerability and susceptibility. The ultimate objective of such an approach must be enhanced resilience of livelihood systems to the epidemic.

de Waal, A. (2003) *'New variant famine': hypothesis, evidence and implications.* Addis Ababa: Commission for HIV/AIDS and Governance in Africa/Economic Commission for Africa.

de Waal, A. and A. **Whiteside** (2003) ''New Variant Famine': AIDS and Food Crisis in Southern Africa', *The Lancet* **362**, pp. 1234-1237.

The paper argues that the recent food crisis in southern Africa is distinct from conventional drought induced food shortages in terms of the profile of those who are vulnerable to starvation as well as in its trajectory of impoverishment and recovery. It is alleged that these new aspects of the food crisis can be attributed largely to the role played by the generalised HIV/AIDS epidemic in the region. Four factors are discussed as being new in this 'new variant famine': household-level labour shortages due to adult morbidity and mortality and a resulting increase in the numbers of dependents; loss of assets and skills due to prime adult mortality; the burden of care for sick adults and children orphaned by AIDS; and the vicious interactions between malnutrition and HIV. It is argued that the way in which HIV/AIDS accentuates existing difficulties such as drought and macro-economic disparities and mismanagement will lead to food insecurity or food emergency becoming a structural feature of the southern African landscape unless countered by innovative intervention strategies (see also de Waal, 2003).

de Waal, A. and J. **Tumushabe** (2003) *HIV/AIDS and Food Security in Africa.* DFID.
http://www.sarpn.org.za/documents/d0000235/P227_AIDS_Food_Security.pdf.

This paper summarises existing evidence concerning HIV/AIDS and food security in sub-Saharan Africa. The two major issues discussed are the impact of HIV/AIDS on agrarian livelihoods and how this impact can be mitigated; and the wider implications of a concurrent generalised HIV/AIDS epidemic and episodes of acute food insecurity, what has been called 'new variant famine'. Concerning the first issue, the paper brings together the evidence from the small-scale studies carried out mainly in eastern, southern and central Africa from the late 1980s onwards which is presented as general knowledge as it is in much of the literature. Additionally, the 'new variant famine' hypothesis is introduced, which posits that many high prevalence African countries who are facing an acute food crisis triggered by drought, floods, low commodity prices, liberalisation of services, mismanagement of food reserves and so forth cannot expect a return to either sustainable livelihoods or a demographic equilibrium, as the adverse impacts of these factors are compounded by HIV/AIDS (for more discussion on the 'new variant famine' hypothesis see de Waal, 2003; de Waal & Whiteside, 2003; for a critique see Ellis, 2003).

Drimie, S. (2002a) 'The Impact of HIV/AIDS on Rural Households and Land Issues in Southern and Eastern Africa'. A Background Paper prepared for the FAO Sub-Regional Office for Southern and Eastern Africa.
http://www.sarpn.org.za/documents/d0000152/index.php.

This background paper summarises key issues surrounding the impact of HIV/AIDS at the rural household level in southern and eastern Africa. It includes sub-sections on general impact in sub-Saharan Africa; underlying causes of the epidemic; economic impact; and impact on household livelihood strategies. From the reviewed literature, serious implications for land-based livelihoods are predicted, as prolonged illness and early death of productive household members alter social relations. An analysis of the impact of HIV/AIDS on land rights or the command positions held by people of different age and gender over land is advocated, which is in effect an analysis of changes in social institutions in which rights to land are anchored (see also Drimie, 2002b).

Drimie, S. (2002b) 'The Impact of HIV/AIDS on Land: Case studies from Kenya, Lesotho and South Africa'. A Synthesis Report prepared for the Southern African Regional Office of the FAO.
http://www.sarpn.org.za/documents/d0000147/P143_Impact_of_HIVAI
DS.pdf.

This paper examines the impact of HIV/AIDS on land issues predominately conceptualised through the lens of the rural household, using case studies from Kenya, Lesotho and South Africa. Land issues are understood to include three main dimensions, namely land use, land rights, and land tenure administration. In addition to findings reported elsewhere concerning land use - most notably land remaining fallow, a switch to less labour intensive crops, a preference for home gardens and an increase in the sale of livestock - the impact of HIV/AIDS on land tenure policies and the functioning of land administration systems is investigated. Special attention is paid to land rights of women and children as well as inheritance practices and norms. After a detailed discussion of each country case study in relation to land use, land rights and land administration, some preliminary policy recommendations are given for each of these three areas. Among those recommendations is the creation of more formalized land tenure policies in order to protect women's and children's legal rights.

Drinkwater, M. (2003) 'HIV/AIDS and Agrarian Change in Southern Africa'. Presentation for the United Nations Regional Inter-Agency Coordination and Support Office Technical Consultation on Vulnerability in the Light of an HIV/AIDS Pandemic, 9-11 September 2003, Johannesburg, South Africa.

This paper proposes what is defined as 'cluster analysis' for want of a better term to understand the dynamics of social change (for a definition of 'cluster' as it is used here see Drinkwater, 1994). Referring to livelihood analyses conducted in Zambia and Zimbabwe, is it argued that cluster analysis techniques with respect to the impact of HIV/AIDS on rural livelihoods show clearly the impact of illness and death amongst urban residents on rural households, an impact that household based analysis often overlooks. More generally, particularly for the analysis of HIV/AIDS impact on rural livelihoods cluster analysis is propagated, as such impact is experienced twofold, in terms of the deterioration of household economies as well as in the unravelling of the social fabric of the lives of those affected or afflicted by AIDS (see also Ellis, 2003, for a discussion of the household and its definition as unit of analysis).

---

du Guerny, J. (2002) *Agriculture and HIV/AIDS.* New York: UNDP.

The paper outlines strategies for the agricultural sector in areas of high HIV/AIDS prevalence. It argues that the agricultural sector should not attempt to carry out health work for which it is ill equipped, but concentrate on agricultural problems, an area where it has a comparative advantage. The discussion is placed into what is called a development framework, which goes beyond the prevailing health framework which dominates the scope of HIV/AIDS strategies and programmes. Two levels of intervention for agricultural policies and programmes are identified: the farming system level, and the farm-household system level. Types of interventions recommended for the agricultural sector at both levels are briefly discussed, as well as how such interventions could dovetail with activities of the health sector.

Engh, I.-E., L. **Stloukal** and J. **du Guerny** (2000) *HIV/AIDS in Namibia: The impact on the livestock sector.* Rome: FAO. http://www.fao.org/sd/wpdirect/WPan0046.htm.

This study is based on the review of literature and field data from two communal area farming regions in Namibia, Oshana and Caprivi. Both regions had at the time of the study the highest HIV infection rates in Namibia. Mixed farming based on crops and livestock is the prevailing farming system, with the latter often representing the predominant source of agricultural income. The study shows HIV/AIDS impact on livestock along similar lines as documented for predominately crop based agricultural systems. The specific effect on livestock is related, as in those systems, to a loss of labour within households accompanied by increased financial expenses. Both these factors lead, among other things, to decreased management of livestock resources and a reduction in draught power due to the sale or slaughter of livestock, the latter in turn affecting crop production.

Additionally, the epidemic has serious effects on the veterinary service and thus on the ability to contain or eliminate livestock diseases. The study also shows a strong gender component in determining impact: The HIV/AIDS afflicted case study households are grouped into three categories: those where husbands had died, those where wives had died, and those where both parents had died. In Oshana in cases were husbands died widespread loss of livestock by the surviving widow and children are the norm (even though there is legislation in place to prevent such 'asset-grapping'); in contrast, in cases where the wife died, a notable lack of disruption of production resources and loss of assets has been observed. In cases were both parents died, an inability of the child headed households to produce enough food seems the norm. In Caprivi, wife inheritance is common and provides a security mechanism for surviving widows and their children. The data also shows that death of an adult (man or women) typically results in households failing to produce enough food due to a reduction in cropped areas, leading to a sale of livestock as a coping mechanism with longer term consequences. Overall, the study highlights the fact that inheritance systems in Namibia are highly complex and the cases discussed are meant to serve mainly as an illustration of the diversity of linkages between HIV/AIDS, property and livestock within these different systems.

Food and Agriculture Organisation of the UN (FAO) - Integrated Support to Sustainable Development and Food Security (IP) Programme (2003) *HIV/AIDS and agriculture: impacts and responses. Case studies from Namibia, Uganda and Zambia.* Rome: FAO.

The three case studies - based on survey and qualitative interview data - discussed in this report demonstrate how different aspects of the HIV/AIDS pandemic affect rural livelihoods in terms of having serious implications for rural agricultural production, household food security, gender concerns, and the policy environment. The case of Uganda shows that AIDS-afflicted households in three different livelihood contexts (mixed agriculture, fisheries, and pastoralist communities) are becoming increasingly resource poor and are producing less; as such they find it increasingly difficult to follow the goals of the Plan for the Modernization of Agriculture implemented by the Ugandan government. The focus in Namibia is on the asset base of widow-headed households. Findings show such households characterised by the dispossession of property following the death of a spouse - even though legislation is in place to protect widows, the capacity to enforce it is lacking. Finally, the case of Zambia shows a steep increase in households fostering orphans. Particularly female headed households are caring for an increasing number of orphans even though they in general have fewer resources available to them than male-headed households. For all three cases, suggestions on how to mitigate the different impacts of HIV/AIDS are made, including mainstreaming HIV/AIDS, developing multi-sectoral responses and creating social protection systems (for the latter see also Devereux, 2003).

Food Economy Group (2002a) *Household food security & HIV/AIDS: Exploring the Linkages.* www.fews.net: Food Economy Group.

The paper describes HIV/AIDS as both, a cause and consequence of food insecurity. It is discussed how the way HIV/AIDS affects rural food security varies over time, as a function of the extent and progression of the disease, as well as over space, due to differences in the ability of households and communities to mitigate the negative effects. In turn, specific livelihood strategies pursued to achieve food security might increase the risk of contracting HIV/AIDS. The paper takes a critical look at the majority of studies on HIV/AIDS impact on food security who tend to focus on the projected effects of household labour reductions on agricultural production. Citing evidence from studies conducted at the household level in Kenya it is argued that the poorest economically active households tend to rely more directly on cash income to secure food than agricultural production, thus a change in employment opportunities might be the major constraint of such households (for a graphic presentation of these studies, see the following reference).

Food Economy Group (2002b) *Food Economy Analysis and the effects of HIV/AIDS on food security at the household level.* www.fews.net: Food Economy Group.

Fox, M., S. **Rosen**, W. **MacLeod**, M. **Wasunna**, M. **Bii**, G. **Foglia** and J. **Simon** (2004) 'The impact of HIV/AIDS on labour productivity in Kenya', *Tropical Medicine and International Health* **9**, pp. 318-324.

This paper reports the results of a study investigating the impact of HIV/AIDS on labour productivity on an agricultural tea estate in Kericho, western Kenya, and describes the 'natural history' of productivity decline associated with AIDS. A retrospective cohort design was used to study the productivity and attendance of tea estate workers who had died or were medically retired because of AIDS-related causes between 1997 and 2002 in comparison with workers perceived as healthy. Comparisons between case and control were made on four measures of productivity: work output (amount of tea leaves plucked) per day; number of days of paid and unpaid leave; number of days of light duty; and total earnings of the individual worker. The results show stable differences in amount plucked per day between case and comparison pluckers and thus a drop in income for the former; during their last three years of life, pluckers who ultimately died of AIDS related causes were absent from work almost twice as often as the comparison workers; in addition, many of the former were shifted to light, on average lower paid duties as they could not carry out plucking activities any longer. Overall impact on productivity as reported in this study might be underestimated as sick workers often bring 'helpers', usually family members, to the field to help with plucking activities, thus supporting their income levels as long as possible.

Gillespie, S. (1989) 'Potential Impact of AIDS on farming systems. A case study from Rwanda', *Land Use Policy* **6**, pp. 301-312.

This early article on AIDS and agriculture assesses the potential impact of HIV/AIDS on farming systems in Rwanda. Two epidemiologically based projection models of the spread of HIV/AIDS are used to predict the proportion of households losing a productive member over the coming ten years. The projected AIDS mortality rates of different age groups are then related to the different levels, type and timing of their respective labour inputs in each type of farming system. Five farming systems within Rwanda are subsequently ranked with respect to their relative sensitivities to the loss of labour through AIDS mortality. While this article is based on early projections, the proposed classification of farming systems according to their vulnerability to labour loss induced by the epidemic is to this day one of the most useful classifications on the level of rural production systems. It has been expanded on by Barnett and Blaikie (1992), and there is much scope for further use in different geographical settings and for different farming systems.

Haddad, L. and S. **Gillespie** (2001a) 'Effective Food and Nutrition Policy Responses to HIV/AIDS: What we know and what we need to know', *Journal of International Development* **13**, pp. 487-511.

This paper addresses the question how government policies in the area of food security, nutrition, agriculture and the environment should be altered to better meet the needs of the poor within the context of the HIV/AIDS epidemic. The relevant literature on HIV/AIDS and rural livelihoods is reviewed, before public policy options for effective mitigation strategies in the areas of agriculture and nutrition are discussed. In addition, the role research can (and should) play in stimulating effective action for AIDS mitigation and ultimately HIV prevention is discussed. Among the priorities for the future the need to include HIV/AIDS in agriculture, food, and nutrition policy is advocated, as well as an integration of the lessons learned and the methodological tools used in investigating impacts of and responses to other shocks within HIV/AIDS impact and mitigation literature. An extended version of this article was published beforehand as a discussion paper, see the following reference.

Haddad, L. and S. **Gillespie** (2001b) *Effective Food and Nutrition Policy Responses to HIV/AIDS: What we know and what we need to know.* Washington DC: International Food Policy Research Institute (IFPRI). http://www.ifpri.org/divs/fcnd/dp/papers/fcndp112.pdf.

Haslwimmer, M. (1996) 'AIDS and Agriculture in sub-Saharan Africa'. http://www.fao.org/waicent/faoinfo/sustdev/WPdirect/WPre0003.htm.

This paper discusses the now well-established impact of HIV/AIDS on rural households, dividing this impact into direct cost (mainly medical and funeral expenses) and indirect cost (those related to the loss of labour). It provides a short general summary of most of the relevant issues concerning agriculture and HIV/AIDS in sub-Saharan Africa without referring to any examples in particular.

International Fund for Agricultural Development (IFAD) (2001) *Strategy Paper On HIV/AIDS For East and Southern Africa*. Rome: IFAD.

The paper starts from the observation that HIV/AIDS has a disproportionate impact on the agricultural sector in having caused the decimation of skilled and unskilled agricultural labour; a reduction in smallholder production; a decline in commercial agriculture; the loss of indigenous farming methods, intergenerational knowledge and specialised skills and practices; and capacity erosion and disruption in the service delivery of formal and informal rural institutions. As a future strategy for an effective response to the epidemic an 'HIV/AIDS vulnerability and mitigation matrix' is proposed as a planning tool as well as the application of an 'HIV and development lens' across sectors within a multisectoral framework of response.

Joling, M. (1996) *AIDS in the family: 'It's just like that.' A study on households coping with AIDS*. Wageningen University, Department of Household and Consumer Science.

This Master's dissertation looks at the way households cope with the HIV/AIDS epidemic in Soroti district in Uganda. As the main problems of afflicted households the following are identified: a high demand for care, leading to less agricultural work performed in the field and longer hours for the care giving women; a decline in the cultivation of land; and a reduction in cash income as less agricultural surplus is produced, leading eventually to the sale of other assets and, as a last resort, to children being taken out of school. Women are identified as the main actors in coping and caring when the epidemic hits the household, but they are found to be less likely to get support when they fall ill themselves. As such, this is one more study confirming trends observed elsewhere.

Kwaramba, P. (1998) *Socio-economic Impact of HIV/AIDS on Communal Agricultural Production and Food Security in Zimbabwe*. FES Working Papers. Harare, Zimbabwe: Friedrich Ebert Stiftung (FES).

This report sets out to assess the impact of HIV/AIDS on communal agriculture in Zimbabwe. It is based largely on data from a questionnaire survey among 544 households in two purposefully selected provinces: Manicaland due to its agricultural diversity, and Mashonaland West, regarded as the breadbasket of the country. In both provinces, two districts are covered. What makes this study particularly interesting is the fact that illness and death due to HIV/AIDS within a household is compared to the situation of households with (illness and) death due to other causes. Main findings include that while all households in which a death occurred suffered a decline in agricultural output, households with AIDS victims registered a statistically significant greater decline in marketed output of maize and cotton. The significant difference in maize (Zimbabwe's main staple crop) signals a threat to household and national food security; a permanent drop in cotton output could lead to agro-industries facing raw material shortages in the future. Interestingly, all households, whether AIDS afflicted or not, reported as their main problem the shortage of inputs and draft power, while labour shortage was regarded by very few households as the major constraint. Concerning marketing of agricultural produce, the report finds that in households where the male head had died, the spouse (or a son) takes over marketing; thus a change in gender relations is said to take place (this change does, however, not affect daughters, who remain sidelined in these matters). Lastly, social ties are reported to be weak. A number of instances are reported where community members take advantage of a household's grief; households who experienced a death, whether AIDS related or not, expect more help from the central government than from local or communal institutions.

Loevinsohn, M. and S. **Gillespie** (2003) *HIV/AIDS, Food Security and Rural Livelihoods: Understanding and Responding*. Washington DC: Regional Network on HIV/AIDS, Rural Livelihoods and Food Security in sub-Saharan Africa (RENEWAL).
http://www.isnar.cgiar.org/renewal/pdf/RENEWALWP2.pdf.

This paper focuses on the interactions between food and nutrition security and HIV/AIDS, and their implications for mitigation strategies. Access to food is seen as fundamental in determining people's choices, and the consequences of AIDS induced illness and death at household and communal level are shaped by features of agricultural and livelihood systems as well as pre-existing patterns of food insecurity. HIV is described as being endogenous to livelihood systems, which are shaped by human actions at many levels from the micro to the macro environment. Policies and programmes affect and influence, positively or negatively, people's susceptibility to HIV or their vulnerability to AIDS' consequences. A major role in responding to the epidemic is envisaged for the agricultural sector, as the need to secure adequate food is the first priority of many afflicted people. More generally, it is argued that there is an urgent need to better understand the pathways along which HIV/AIDS moves through societies. To arrive at such an understanding, the use of an 'HIV/AIDS lens' is advocated - conceptualised as a tool for reviewing development actions from the perspective of the evolving knowledge of AIDS interactions.

Menon, R., M. **Wawer**, J. **Konde-Lule**, N. **Sewankambo** and C. **Li** (1998) 'The economic impact of adult mortality on households in Rakai district, Uganda', in M. Ainsworth, L. Fransen and M. Over (eds.) *Confronting AIDS: Evidence from the Developing World, selected background papers for the World Bank Policy Research Report Confronting AIDS: Public Priorities in a Global Epidemic*, pp. 325-339. Luxembourg: Office for Official Publications of the European Commission.

This study assesses the economic impact of adult mortality on households in Rakai district in south-western Uganda, using longitudinal survey information regarding adult mortality in households between 1989 and 1992. An interesting aspect of the study is that comparisons are made between households where at least one of the death was of an HIV-positive adult and households where none of the death was of an HIV-positive adult. A decline in resources and economic status - defined in this study by the ownership of durable goods - occurred only in households were the adult death was of an HIV-positive individual, a fact that occurred even when the adults who died were of an equivalent age range (15-50 years). Another factor determining whether household economic status declined was the gender of the individual who died. Households where the diseased was male were more likely to suffer a reduction in ownership of durable goods than households were the diseased was female.

Mongi, R. (2002) *Assessment of the Impact of HIV/AIDS Epidemic on the Coffee-Banana Farming System in Arumeru District, Tanzania.* Larenstein University of Professional Education.

This is an interesting case study of the impact of HIV/AIDS on households within this particular farming system. Similar to other smallholder systems, labour is identified as the limiting factor for increased production, and thus the loss of labour due to the epidemic has a direct impact on farming activities. While the gender division of labour within this farming system is described as dynamic, it are nevertheless men who have control over the activities which provide the most significant sources of income and women who are required to carry out additional tasks arising as the epidemic progresses. Field extension offices in Arumeru in fact report the loss of women's labour due to care duties as a main constraint in agricultural activities. Two diagrams of a small holder farm in this coffee-banana system, one before and one after the HIV/AIDS epidemic, illustrate its impact on a household within the system.

Morton, J. (2003) 'Conceptualising the links between HIV/AIDS and pastoralist livelihoods'. Paper presented at the Annual Conference of the Development Studies Association, 10 - 12 September 2003, Glasgow.

While the understanding of the links between HIV/AIDS and agriculture based livelihoods is increasing, there has been virtually no research on the links between HIV/AIDS and pastoralism. This paper thus identifies key potential linkages between HIV/AIDS and pastoralism by combining conceptual frameworks from the literature on HIV/AIDS and agriculture - in particular the concepts of susceptibility versus resistance to HIV infection, and vulnerability versus resilience to the impacts of AIDS - with an understanding of core common features as well as the diversity of pastoralist livelihoods.

In doing so, it provides a good overview over all potentially relevant themes and identifies future research priorities.

National Agricultural Advisory Service (NAADS) (2003) *The impact of HIV/AIDS on the agricultural sector and rural livelihoods in Uganda.* Uganda: NAADS.

This study provides an in-depth analysis of the non-health effects of HIV/AIDS on individuals, different household types and communities within the mixed agriculture, fisheries, and pastoral subsectors in parts of Uganda. It is based on a survey of smallholder agricultural rural households at six sites in the Lake Victoria Crescent agro-ecological zone who were asked to provide comparative data for the period from 1997 to 2002. Within all three subsectors, most households were found to depend mainly on asset sales to meet the cost of HIV/AIDS related illness or death. Other major findings - apart from the often reported dynamics of reduced agricultural output and reductions in herd size, and a shift from labour intensive to low-labour input activities, all contributing to decreased income and food security - include an observed shifting in gender roles among in particular mixed agriculture and pastoral communities, and an emergence of new communal institutions while at the same time traditional support networks have often collapsed. Even though data on the pastoral communities was more difficult to come by, findings indicate that this is the community most vulnerable to the impact of the epidemic. Coping strategies as devised by afflicted households are discussed and classified into three categories: labour-related, nutrition-related, and income related. Based on these observed coping mechanisms, the report ends with further recommendations to mitigate the effects of the epidemic.

Opoyi, P. (2001) *HIV/AIDS, Gender and Livelihood in Siaya District, Kenya. An Analysis of AIDS Impact on Rural Households.* Wageningen University.

This thesis provides a good example of the importance of gender issues in considering HIV/AIDS impact in general and impact on (rural) livelihoods in particular. The district in the centre of this study can be described as a labour reserve for urban industries. Household livelihood strategies thus centre on men working in town and sending remittances whenever possible, whereas women stay behind and are engaged in agricultural production or other income earning activities, including commercial sex work. In terms of HIV/AIDS, Siaya district is thus a highly susceptible environment. The Luo society in the study area is further characterised by a lack of elasticity of gender roles, which makes it difficult for households to adapt to the changes in household gender profiles brought about by AIDS related illness and death. Findings include that among low-income households, those headed by widows or other women adapt more easily and develop more sustainable coping strategies than those headed by men.

Qamar, M. (2001) 'The HIV/AIDS epidemic: An unusual challenge to agricultural extension services in sub-Saharan Africa', *Journal of Agricultural Education* **8**, pp. 1-11.

The starting point for this article is the observation that the loss of breadwinners due to the epidemic is leading to increased poverty and food insecurity among many afflicted households in sub-Saharan Africa, while professionals, including agricultural extension workers, have not been spared by the epidemic. Impact is thus felt at household level as well as at the level of relevant (agricultural) organisations and institutions. This situation created by the epidemic asks for a review of approaches, methodologies, and technologies in agricultural extension service provision in order to take account of the new clientele for extension services, for example women and young people. However, most countries in sub-Saharan Africa are without a clear policy on agricultural extension in general, let alone a policy on HIV/AIDS and extension services in particular.

Rugalema, G. (1999) *Adult Mortality as Entitlement Failure. AIDS and the Crisis of Rural Livelihoods in a Tanzanian Village.* The Hague: Institute of Social Studies (ISS).

Rugalema's study provides a detailed analysis of the impact of HIV/AIDS on the Buhaya Livelihood in Bukoba district in Tanzania. His central argument is that in order to understand the relationship between increased prime adult mortality due to AIDS and the livelihoods of rural households, one needs to relate the changing demographic structure to the changing assets portfolio of those households. On one hand, AIDS induced morbidity and mortality has far-reaching consequences for households due to its adverse effect on the availability of labour and a depletion of productive assets. At the same time, it leads to changes in household composition particularly regarding the gender and age balance, changes which in turn are shown to adversely affect a household's ability to reorganise its livelihood and in the longer term potentially lead to changes in the farming system. The study is an excellent example of the impacts of HIV/AIDS on rural households, livelihoods and the farming system in one particular community at a particular point in time - a point in time when AIDS induced mortality was highest among prime male adults. While this epidemiological trend seems to have been reversed, the study still serves as a good example for studying the impact of HIV/AIDS on rural households and communities as a dynamic and systematic process.

Rugalema, G. with S. **Weigang** and J. **Mbwika** (1999) *HIV/AIDS and the Commercial Agricultural Sector of Kenya*. Rome: FAO.

This report presents an analysis of the relationship between excess morbidity and mortality due to HIV/AIDS and the commercial viability of the commercial agricultural sector of Kenya. The analysis is based on data from five agro-estates in altogether three provinces (Nyanza, Rift Valley and Eastern Kenya), all of which feel the impact of HIV/AIDS but to different degrees. Main findings include that due to HIV related illness agro-estates face rising cost and losses in profits due to a loss of workers and working hours. Medical and funeral expenses exceed budget provisions, and terminal benefits, retraining and replacement measures add further to the expenses incurred by the epidemic. Labour intensive companies, such as sugar estates, which in addition heavily depend on out-growers (individual farmers who supply cane to the estate) are particularly hard hit, as cultivation patterns of some afflicted out-growers change to the less labour intensive agricultural production of cassava and maize. At the same time, on all surveyed estates social, economic and environmental factors are common which favour the spread of the epidemic, including poor housing, overcrowding, lack of recreational facilities, and unequal income earning opportunities for men and women. The report ends with a number of recommendation on how to prevent further socio-economic effects of the epidemic and to mitigate its current impact.

Shah, M., N. **Osborne**, T. **Mbilizi** and G. **Vilili** (2002) *Impact of HIV/AIDS on Agricultural Productivity and Rural Livelihoods in the Central Region of Malawi.* CARE International Malawi.

This detailed study based on participatory research methods gives a good overview over the potentially debilitating impact of HIV/AIDS on farming households in particular and rural production systems in general, exemplified using the example of three districts in central Malawi. Household level analysis is embedded into an analysis of existing social relations and livelihood strategies within the study villages. The study confirms findings reported elsewhere: Chronic sickness (this term was used by the fieldwork team in order to avoid the sensitive issue of naming HIV/AIDS directly) tends to trigger a sequence of impacts on the rural household economy, the most immediate of which is loss of labour, leading to decreased agricultural productivity. Other findings include that impact varies considerably due to the timing of sickness or death in the household and its relation to the agricultural cycle, the duration of the sickness, multiple stresses a household experiences, and relative economic status of a household. Social norms of marriage were another factor that determined the type of impact, for example women in patrilocal villages were found to be more vulnerable than women in matrilocal villages (both types existed in the study areas), as the latter continue to use their own land even after remarriage. The main source of support for rural households was found to come from kinship networks. In general, people were more willing to help richer households in order to possibly earn themselves a favour to be redeemed in the future. The data also shows that the impact of chronic sickness is not just felt within the nuclear household where it occurs, but often impacts several households within the kinship network (giving rise to questioning the adequacy of the household as category of analysis, see also Drinkwater, 1994 and 2003, on the 'cluster').

Southern African Development Community (SADC) Food, Agriculture and Natural Resources (FANR) Vulnerability Assessment Committee (2003) *Towards Identifying Impacts of HIV/AIDS on Food Insecurity in Southern Africa and Implications for Response. Findings from Malawi, Zambia and Zimbabwe.* Harare: SADC FANR.

The paper starts from the assumption that HIV/AIDS has contributed to the problems faced by rural households in southern Africa in the context of the 2002 food emergency. It aims to show the extent of that contribution and how it varies according to the demographic structure, as well as the mortality and morbidity profiles of households. It does so by using data generated from the emergency food security assessments conducted in Malawi, Zambia and Zimbabwe in 2002 to study the relationship between HIV/AIDS proxy variables and food security parameters. Findings include that the presence or absence of a healthy adult aged between 18 and 59 as household head has more pronounced effects on household food security than does the dependency ratio, while the general presence of a chronically ill person (other than the head) does not have a strong negative effect on food security. This raises questions concerning indicators for targeted interventions. The study argues that where households are found to have experienced a decline in income and agricultural production due to HIV/AIDS, there is a need for continued consumption-oriented assistance in the form of safety net programmes, even after immediate food emergencies have passed. Overall, to address HIV/AIDS mitigation a 'three-pronged attack' is advocated: in addition to consumption side support this should include productivity enhancing support (an example includes Farmer Life Schools pioneered in South East Asia), and support to household and community safety nets. Policy needs to be reviewed through an 'HIV/AIDS lens' (see also Loevinsohn & Gillespie, 2003).

Stokes, S. (2003) *Measuring Impacts of HIV/AIDS on Rural Livelihoods and Food Security.* Rome: FAO.
http://www.fao.org/sd/2003/PE0102a_en.htm.

This paper uses the sustainable livelihoods framework in the development of indicators to measure the impacts of HIV/AIDS on rural households and food security. Each of the five capital assets - human, financial, natural, social and physical capital - is demonstrated to be impacted by the epidemic. Human capital impacts are being identified as central to measure effects of the epidemic, because declines in human capital are said to reverberate throughout other capital assets. By focusing measurements on those assets rural households are believed to use to sustain their livelihoods, potential areas for mitigation efforts can be identified.

Tibaijuka, A. (1997) 'AIDS and Economic Welfare in Peasant Agriculture: Case Studies from Kagabiro Village, Kagera Region, Tanzania', *World Development* **25**, pp. 963-975.

This paper presents a review of the progression of the AIDS epidemic in Tanzania in general and Kagera region in particular related to cultural, economic and institutional factors. These factors are identified as a culture that inherently encourages multiple sexual relationships; a high risk of infection due to inadequate health services; and continued economic decline and lack of worthwhile alternatives which has increased the rate of migration and sex work. This is followed by a case study which quantifies the impact of AIDS on the economic welfare of households and a village community. The case discussed is the village of Kagabiro in Muleba district, some 70 kilometres from Bukoba town along one of the country's main trunk roads. Findings show that the adverse impact of AIDS on household and community welfare has been considerable due to production foregone as labour is reallocated to nurse and mourn victims; declining farm productivity as assets and working capital are sold to pay medical bills; and rising dependency burdens. To bring the epidemic under control the study recommends research into community-based strategies which can foster new social ethics; promote rural productivity and employment; improve health services; and provide safety nets for survivor's families.

Topouzis, D. (1998) *The Implications of HIV/AIDS for Rural Development Policy and Programming: Focus on sub-Saharan Africa*. Rome: FAO and UNDP.

This paper examines the interrelationship between rural development and HIV/AIDS in sub-Saharan Africa. This relationship is bi-directional in the sense that the epidemic may have an effect on formal and informal rural institutions, while at the same time policies and programmes of rural institutions may facilitate or contain the spread of the epidemic. Overall, causes and consequences of the HIV epidemic are regarded as closely related with wider challenges to development: HIV/AIDS tends to exacerbate existing development problems through its catalytic effects and systematic impact. The paper proposes a conceptual framework with a focus on five areas crucial to rural development for the identification of the main policy and programming issues raised by the epidemic. These are poverty alleviation; food security and sustainable livelihoods; empowerment of rural women; labour; and infrastructure. As one important aspect the interplay between food and livelihood security on one hand, and rural women's agency on the other is discussed.

Topouzis, D. (1999) *The Implications of HIV/AIDS for Household Food Security in Africa*. Addis Abeba: United Nations Economic Commission for Africa, Food Security and Sustainable Development Division.

The paper analyses some of the linkages between HIV/AIDS, gender, and household food security in rural Africa. It is argued that the adverse effects of HIV/AIDS morbidity and mortality on rural households may disrupt the interface between productive and domestic labour. Rural women as food producers, custodians of household food security and caregivers are at the centre of that interface. Thus gender may play a key role in determining both, the impact of HIV/AIDS on household food security and the ability of a household to cope with it. A useful graphic representation shows how HIV/AIDS has a systematic effect on household food security, disrupting not only certain aspects of food security, but the entire food system. Another graphic outlines household food security coping strategies, their impact on household resources, and their degree of reversibility. Some of these strategies, however, may disintegrate shortly after prime male adult death, as widows' claims to household assets might not be secured. One coping mechanism to food insecurity for women is sex, but very little is known systematically about this type of exchange as a coping mechanism to food insecurity, even though it is an area central to women's reproductive health. In general it is argued that small differences in terms of more equitable gender roles within households and communities can have a positive impact on food security in households afflicted by the epidemic.

Topouzis, D. (2000) *Measuring the Impact of HIV/AIDS on the Agricultural Sector in Africa*. Geneva: UNAIDS Best Practice Collection.

This background paper takes as its starting point that agriculture is the mainstay of many African economies, but that the adverse effects of the HIV/AIDS epidemic in particular on smallholder agriculture are often too subtle to be visible at macro-level. There thus is a need to systematically monitor the impact on the agricultural sector, beyond the isolated impact studies undertaken to date which are no longer enough to shape adequate political responses. The paper gives examples how this can be achieved. The ultimate objective of such monitoring is to make rural households and communities dependent on (subsistence) agriculture more resilient to the evolving HIV/AIDS epidemics. Strategies proposed to help strengthening those communities' capacity to cope will, it is argued, need to encompass gender policies, food security policies, and shifts from production-oriented policies to livelihood-oriented ones. Livelihood Vulnerability Mapping is advocated as a tool for monitoring impact as well as designing mitigation programmes.

Topouzis, D. (2003) *Addressing the Impact of HIV/AIDS on Ministries of Agriculture: Focus on Eastern and Southern Africa*. Rome: FAO. http://www.fao.org/hivaids/publications/moa.pdf.

This study is based on the assumption that Ministries of Agriculture (MoAs) can be instrumental in mitigating the effects of HIV/AIDS. It examines the relevance of HIV/AIDS to MoAs and their work in relation to smallholder agriculture in eastern and southern Africa. The four areas of HIV/AIDS impact analysed in detail are: MoA staff vulnerability to HIV infection and AIDS impact; disruption of MoA operations and capacity erosion; increased vulnerability of MoA clients to food and livelihood insecurity; and the relevance of MoA programmes in view of the conditions created by HIV/AIDS. A MoA response to the epidemic needs to address the impact of HIV/AIDS within the ministry; and adjust agricultural policies, strategies and programmes to the adverse effects created by the epidemic. Among the findings are a need to generically include awareness raising into all core activities of the ministry; a need to introduce HIV/AIDS into the budget of MoAs (which at the time of writing had only just happened in Uganda); a need to shift from the prevailing production-oriented approaches to agricultural and rural development towards a client based approach in which MoA programmes reflect the evolving needs, constraints and living conditions of their clients (this is not only necessary in the light of HIV/AIDS impact but more generally, but becomes more urgent in the face of HIV/AIDS). More broadly, the need is advocated to incorporate the developmental implications of HIV/AIDS into core agricultural policies, strategies and programmes, which requires a shift towards a developmental paradigm of response that complements health-based with core agricultural initiatives.

Topouzis, D. with G. **Hemrich** (1994) *The Socio-Economic Impact of HIV and AIDS on Rural Families in Uganda: An Emphasis on Youth*. Study Paper No. 2. New York: UNDP.
http://www.undp.org/hiv/publications/study/english/sp2e.htm.

This study investigating the impact of HIV/AIDS on rural families with a special focus on Youth (defined as three distinct groups, namely children, adolescents, and young adults, ranging from 10 to 25 years of age) was carried out in 1993 in the three Ugandan districts of Kabarole, Tororo and Gulu by research teams including an international consultant on HIV/AIDS and local counterparts. Methods used included Rapid Rural Appraisal and Participatory Rural Appraisal techniques, focus group discussions, in depth interviews with HIV afflicted and affected families and Youth, school visits and Knowledge-Attitude-Practice questionnaire surveys (results of the latter are however not formally incorporated into the study report). The focus on Youth is based on the assumption that Youth are the most vulnerable group to HIV infection but at the same time also the most promising agents for behavioural change.

Main findings of the study (in addition to the more widely observed disruption in extension and other government services due to the high death toll among qualified civil servants and technocrats) include the following: The HIV epidemic follows different pattern in each location. Even two villages in the same district - due to different agro-ecological conditions and customs that determine sexual behaviour and attitudes towards HIV/AIDS - could show radical differences. The epidemic disproportionally affects young rural women, as far more women lost their husbands to AIDS than vice versa. In all three districts an AIDS stigma - built on a prevailing stereotype that women are responsible for transmitting the epidemic - was shown to undermine traditional coping mechanisms which are under 'normal' conditions accessible to young widows, thus changing the socio-economic fabric of the family. The study advocates that for behavioural change to be effective, socio-economic and cultural realities and norms that influence sexual behaviour (including early sexual relations, alcohol and drug use, a widespread bar and disco culture, ritual cleansing and wife inheritance) need to be taken account of when designing interventions. Concerning outreach activities to Youth in particular, the need to differentiate between in-school and out-of-school Youth or school drop-outs (the latter making up the majority of rural young people in the study areas) is emphasised: Especially girls and young women out of school have hardly been reached by any HIV/AIDS intervention activities.

Waller, K. (1997) *The Impact of HIV/AIDS on Farming Households in the Monze District of Zambia*. Bath: University of Bath. http://www.bath.ac.uk/ ~ hssjgc/kate.html.

This informative study of HIV/AIDS impact on farming households in the Monze district of Zambia uses baseline data from a survey conducted in 1991 to analyse how HIV/AIDS undermines household responsiveness to cope with a number of other exogenous shocks that have hit Zambian farmers over the preceding five years, namely agricultural policy reform, years of drought, and death of cattle due to disease. What makes the study particularly interesting are the facts that it uses household case studies as well as Drinkwater's (1994; 2003) representation of 'cluster' to represent relations between households, and the concept of 'hearth-holder' (Bryceson, 1995) to account for female centred relationships between members of different households; additionally it presents detailed household case material in an annex and analyses this material in terms of showing the strain on and partly change in gender divisions due to HIV/AIDS. Households are grouped into five stereotypic types of households according to wealth, agricultural, and demographic characteristics. While the general difficulty of disentangling the impact of HIV/AIDS from the other shocks mentioned above remains, the study overall shows how traditional responses to such shocks have been undercut for HIV/AIDS afflicted and/or affected households by labour shortages coupled with medical or transport expenses, and that HIV/AIDS compounded with other shocks has generally reduced household food security and overall economic productivity.

White, J. and E. **Robinson** (2000) *HIV/AIDS and Rural Livelihoods in sub-Saharan Africa*. Policy Series 6. Greenwich: University of Greenwich, Natural Resources Institute.

This paper discusses most of the literature dealing with the socio-economic impact of HIV/AIDS on rural livelihoods in sub-Saharan Africa and its shortcomings. HIV/AIDS is defined as having a 'bi-directional' relationship with the processes related to development in that it has an impact on the socio-economic dynamics of households and communities, while socio-economic change itself may have a negative or positive impact on the spread of HIV/AIDS. Critical points discussed include: the tendency within the existing literature to generalise from limited base-line data on wider impacts of the epidemic; a failure to recognise the methodological problem of identifying sickness and death due to HIV/AIDS as a single factor affecting local livelihood systems; and a failure apparent in most household-level research on HIV/AIDS to draw on the existing literature on shocks to rural households and coping strategies and thus forgo an opportunity to integrate issues concerning HIV/AIDS with existing generic work. As a way forward the study proposes to revisit some of the original baseline data gathered in the late 1980s and early 1990s to gain a better understanding of the longer term impact of HIV/AIDS within other processes that affect behaviour and contribute to poverty. It is also advocated to shift attention from the household as the focus of analysis and the key entry point for programme intervention towards household- and community-level studies that better track the connections among rural, urban, and peri-urban groups.

Yamano, T. and T. **Jayne** (2004) 'Measuring the Impacts of Working-Age Adult Mortality on Small-Scale Farm Households in Kenya', *World Development* **32**, pp. 91-119.

This study uses a two year panel of 1,422 Kenyan households surveyed in 1997 and 2000 and measures how prime-age adult mortality affects rural households' size and composition, agricultural production, assets levels, and off-farm income. In quantitatively estimating the effects of the disease on farm production and off-farm incomes, it seeks to make a contribution to arrive at reliable macro-level projections of the effects of HIV/AIDS, for which the absence of nationally representative micro-level information remains a critical limitation. Some of the findings are consistent with household coping behaviours as described by qualitative studies in the literature, most notably the importance of dis-aggregating the effects of prime-age adult death by gender, age and status (the role and position of the individual in the household). Results indicate that relatively poor households are unable to recover quickly from the effects of prime-age head-of-household adult mortality, as the effects on crop and non-farm incomes did not diminish over the three year survey interval.

2. HIV/AIDS and broader development issues

Armstrong, J. (1995) *Uganda's AIDS Crisis. Its Implications for Development.* World Bank Discussion Papers No. 298. Washington DC: World Bank.

This paper traces the social and economic channels through which the AIDS epidemic is likely to make its impact on Uganda's development prospects as perceived at the time of writing. In particular, it examines the impact on health expenditure, based on projections of essential drugs that would be needed to treat opportunistic diseases of persons with AIDS. It also looks at the impact of the epidemic on agricultural production from both, household and farming system perspective, and explores the wider ramifications on the labour force. Recommendations and areas for further research conclude the study. While somehow dated, the study still provides a comprehensive overview over the possible relationship between HIV/AIDS and overall societal development in a country with a predominately rural economy, an economy in which women are the main producers of food. Concerning in particular the projected impact of the epidemic on the agricultural sector, later developments have confirmed many of the study's predictions.

Barnett, T., E. **Blas** and A. **Whiteside** (eds) (1996) *AIDS Briefs. Integrating HIV/AIDS into Sectoral Planning.*
http://sara.aed.org.

These AIDS briefs - a joint effort by the World Health Organisation Global Programme on AIDS, the Support for Analysis and Research in Africa Project (SARA), the Health and Human Resources Analysis for Africa (HHRAA) Project and the U.S. Agency for International Development (USAID) Africa Bureau - deal with susceptibility and vulnerability to HIV/AIDS and how these can be reduced covering the following eight areas: commercial agriculture; subsistence agriculture; education; health; manufacturing; mining; tourism; and military populations. For each of these a short summary outlining the impact of the HIV epidemic is given, followed by a vulnerability checklist, possible responses, and a list of useful references.

Barnett, T. and A. **Whiteside** (2002) *AIDS in the Twenty-First Century. Disease and Globalization.* Basingstoke: Palgrave Macmillan.

This book brings together in one place insights from the work of both authors on the HIV/AIDS epidemic and its social and economic impact since the mid 1980s. Situating the epidemic within the wider framework of globalisation and inequality, its three parts discuss comprehensively all the areas HIV/AIDS touches upon. The first part serves as an introduction to the disease and its epidemiology. The second part deals with susceptibility, with a special focus on the roots of the epidemic and a discussion on why to date the African continent bears the major burden. Part three discusses vulnerability and impact, with subsections on individuals, households and communities; orphans and the elderly; subsistence agriculture and rural livelihoods; the private sector; economic growth; governance issues, and possible responses. The book is a good starting point to get an understanding of the epidemic and its nature from where then specific interests can be pursued, aided by its comprehensive bibliography.

Béchu, N. (1998) 'The impact of AIDS on the economy of families in Côte d'Ivoire: Changes in consumption among AIDS-affected households', in M. Ainsworth, L. Fransen and M. Over (eds.) *Confronting AIDS: Evidence from the Developing World, selected background papers for the World Bank Policy Research Report Confronting AIDS: Public Priorities in a Global Epidemic*, pp. 341-348. Luxembourg: Office for Official Publications of the European Commission.

Using data on 200 mostly urban households in Côte d'Ivoire, this survey based study shows how consumption patterns change in AIDS affected households. The main finding is that a substantial fall in consumption expenditures is observed during the first few months following the detection of the illness, while a general upturn is observed a few months later. This relative upturn, however, does not enable households experiencing an AIDS death to return to their earlier levels of consumption. A major weakness of the study is that the unit of analysis is the quasi unitary household: no allowances are made for the fact that expenditure (and recovery) patterns might vary considerably according to the gender of the household member who falls ill.

Devereux, S. (2003) *Policy Options for Increasing the Contribution of Social Protection to Food Security*. Forum for Food Security in Southern Africa. London: Overseas Development Institute (ODI). http://www.odi.org.uk/Food-Security-Forum/Index.html.

This report identifies three sets of factors - HIV/AIDS, market liberalisation, and governance failures - to explain why southern Africa (countries covered include Lesotho, Malawi, Mozambique, Zambia and Zimbabwe) coped less effectively with the food crisis of 2001/2002 than with the previous drought of 1991/1992 and suggests that new needs for social protection might be emerging. Social protection is defined as a mechanism to reduce vulnerability to livelihood shocks. Here a clear distinction has to be made between social assistance to vulnerable individuals unable to make a livelihood, and social insurance to support the working poor against livelihood shocks like droughts or the HIV/AIDS epidemic. The paper advocates an analysis that instead of treating the food crisis as a food emergency at household level regards it as a livelihood crisis at community level, which in turn requires an integrated approach that addresses the underlying causes of vulnerability. Some suggestions are in due course discussed on how to address such vulnerabilities, leading to a discussion of the pros and cons of the Poverty Reduction Strategy Papers (PRSPs) in the respective participating countries. More fundamentally, the question is posed whether increasingly unpredictable harvests may require a radical rethink of the role of family farming as a livelihood strategy for the rural poor in southern Africa.

Ellis, F. (2003) *Human Vulnerability and Food Insecurity: Policy Implications*. Forum for Food Security in Southern Africa. London: Overseas Development Institute (ODI). http://www.odi.org.uk/Food-Security-Forum/Index.html.

This paper reviews vulnerability concepts and relates these to factors implicated in the 2001-2003 food security crisis in southern Africa (countries covered include Lesotho, Malawi, Mozambique, Zambia and Zimbabwe). Vulnerability is defined as a forward looking concept that seeks to describe how prone individuals, households, certain groups, and broader populations are to being unable to cope with adverse events. Factors causing rising vulnerability in southern Africa are identified as growth failures, market liberalisation failures, HIV/AIDS, and politics and governance issues. All factors are given the same relevance, which arguably fails to understand the specific kind of shock HIV/AIDS poses (even though it is acknowledged that traditional famine coping strategies might not be viable in the face of AIDS).

Foreman, M. and F. **Belton** (1992) *The Hidden Cost of AIDS: The Challenge of HIV to Development.* London: Panos Institute.

This comprehensive report is the first of its kind looking at HIV/AIDS primarily as an economic and social issue and discussing its impact on all sectors of society. Its chapters include a general discussion of the HIV pandemic, its modes of transmission and its gender dimension; an overview over the demographic impact; a discussion of health costs as well as social cost, particularly at community level; the impact on labour and human resources; vulnerability of rural households and threats to food security; consequences at national level; a discussion of mitigation strategies; and finally the possible role of development interventions at local, national and global level. Even though the report was produced in 1992, much of what it says is still valid to date and it provides a good overview over the wider issues related to the epidemic (for another such overview see Barnett & Whiteside, 2002).

Mutangadura, G. (2000) 'Household welfare impacts of mortality of adult females in Zimbabwe: Implications for policy and program development'. Paper presented at The AIDS and Economics Symposium, organised by the International AIDS Economics Network (IAEN), Durban, 7-8 July 2000.

Looking at women as gatekeepers to household food security and key players in the overall household economy, the paper investigates the welfare impact of female mortality at household level in Manicaland province of Zimbabwe. Two sites were selected for this study, an urban site and a rural site. Findings indicate that the major household welfare impacts of adult female mortality are food insecurity, a decrease in access to school, an increased work burden of children, and loss of assets. Empirical evidence from the research also indicates that elderly women pursuing informal business activities have become the leading foster parents of surviving maternal orphans, and that maternal relatives have become the main carers of orphans - contrary to tradition which demands that paternal relatives be the main source of orphan care. Overall, sixty five percent of households where the deceased adult female used to live before her death were reported to be no longer in existence in both the urban and rural sites. Policy responses which might strengthen the coping capacity of surviving households are suggested and include government support to secure secondary schooling for orphans; support for the elderly; and a strengthening of community initiatives.

Rugalema, G. (2000) 'Coping or Struggling? A Journey into the Impact of HIV/AIDS in Southern Africa', *Review of African Political Economy (ROAPE)* **86**, pp. 537-545.

The article questions the wisdom of employing the notion of coping strategies to analyse the effects of morbidity and mortality associated with HIV/AIDS in rural Africa. It is argued that in areas hard hit by AIDS the concept of coping strategies is of limited value in explaining household experiences and may in fact serve to divert policy-makers from the enormity of the emergency. To say that households are coping implies they are at the very least persevering. Research, however, has shown that adult mortality in a considerable number of cases results in household dissolution, a clear indication of a failure to cope. The conceptual framework built around the notion of coping is derived from famine survival strategies of rural households. Such strategies might be ill suited to analyse household responses to morbidity and mortality associated with HIV/AIDS.

Seeley, J. (2002) 'Thinking with the livelihoods framework in the context of the HIV/AIDS epidemic'.
http://www.livelihoods.org/static/jseeley_NN136.htm.

Using a livelihoods framework, this paper explores how the HIV/AIDS epidemic touches not only human capital in the form of affecting people's health, but all aspects of the lives of those infected as well as of those living in communities affected. The need to look beyond health interventions in mitigating the epidemic is shown by highlighting the impact on financial, economic, social and physical capital as well as looking at the influence of the epidemic on seasonal and other forms of vulnerability and the policy and institutional environment in which livelihoods are constructed and sustained. It is stressed that those living with HIV/AIDS have other and often more pressing concerns than sickness, including to sustain their livelihoods. A contribution that livelihoods approaches can make is that of highlighting the impact of the epidemic in all areas of people's lives and thus help to ensure that when prioritising responses the non-health aspects of the epidemic are not neglected.

Webb, D. and S. **Paquette** (2000) 'The potential role of food aid in mitigating the impacts of HIV/AIDS: the case of Zambia', *Development in Practice* **10**, pp. 694-700.

In taking the example of Zambia, the article starts from the assumption that mitigating the impact of AIDS at household and community level is complicated by the difficulty of isolating such impacts from the more generalised effects of chronic poverty and other adverse conditions such as recurrent drought or structural adjustment policies. Need profiles of chronically ill seem to demonstrate that food provision is of utmost importance to afflicted households. This is due to the fact that when a family member falls ill, the (mostly female) task of acquiring sufficient food is unwillingly given second priority to that of caring for the patient. It is advocated that the dynamics of HIV/AIDS require interventions that are both, health and development oriented, and carefully targeted food aid has an important role to play in both areas. Food aid should in such set-ups be considered not as supplementary feeding, but primarily as a temporary income transfer to afflicted and affected households, and be accompanied by other measures such as training and skill development programmes.

World Bank (1997) *Confronting AIDS. Public Priorities in a Global Epidemic.* Washington, DC: World Bank.

This World Bank Report summarizes the main findings from a detailed study carried out in the high HIV/AIDS prevalence region of Kagera in Tanzania in the early 1990s. It is one of the first major studies linking HIV/AIDS to the whole range of wider development issues. Issues discussed include how widespread poverty and unequal income distribution stimulate the spread of the epidemic; how processes accompanying desirable economic development (accelerated labour migration, urbanisation, and cultural modernisation) at the same time are conducive to the spread of the epidemic; how at household level AIDS deaths exacerbate poverty and social inequality, which in turn fuel the epidemic, thus creating a vicious circle. The report also introduces a typology which classifies country wide epidemics according to two broad criteria (the extent of HIV infection among groups of people engaged in high risk behaviour, and whether the infection has spread to populations assumed to practice low risk behaviour) into nascent, concentrated, or generalized epidemics. As the most cost-effective intervention it is suggested to target high-risk populations (for example commercial sex workers). Additional household survey based impact studies carried out at the same time by World Bank policy research teams include Béchu (1998) in Côte d'Ivoire and Menon et. al. (1998) in Uganda.

3. Other readings

On gender issues in rural settings in sub-Saharan Africa:

Bryceson, D. (1995) *Women Wielding the Hoe. Lessons from Rural Africa for Feminist Theory and Development Practice.* Oxford: Berg Publishers.

Waterhouse, R. and C. **Vijfhuizen** (2001) *Strategic Women, Gainful Men. Gender, land and natural resources in different rural contexts in Mozambique.* Maputo, Mozambique: University of Eduardo Mondlane.

On the 'cluster' as unit of analysis:

Drinkwater, M. (1994) 'Developing interaction and understanding: RRA and farmer research groups in Zambia', in I. Scoones and J. Thompson (eds) *Beyond Farmer First. Rural people's knowledge, agricultural research and extension practice*, pp. 133-139. London: Intermediate Technology Publications.

4. World wide web resources on HIV/AIDS and agriculture in sub-Saharan Africa

The World Wide Web is an important source of information about all issues related to HIV/AIDS.[13] The first calling point for any web search on HIV/AIDS is naturally the homepage of the Joint United Nations Programme on HIV/AIDS (UNAIDS) at http://www.unaids.org. It provides among other things regularly updated epidemiological fact sheets on the state of the epidemic in each country; a bibliographical database and the possibility to download documents; and links to HIV/AIDS related activities of other international organisations.

Some of these organisations in the field of development have meanwhile a special link-page for HIV/AIDS related issues, or can be searched for topical information on such issues. These include the World Bank (WB) at http://www1.worldbank.org/hiv_aids, the World Health Organisation (WHO) at http://www.who.int, the United Nations Development Programme (UNDP) at http://www.undp.org, and the United Nations Research Institute for Social Development (UNRISD) at http://www.unrisd.org.

Looking specifically at HIV/AIDS and agriculture, the following three web-addresses are of particular importance:

Firstly, the website of the United Nations Food and Agricultural Organisation (FAO) at http://www.fao.org, with a link to http://www.fao.org/hivaids/publications/index_en.htm, from where a number of FAO publications on HIV/AIDS and agriculture can be accessed.

Another important source of information is the site of the International Food Policy Research Institute (IFPRI) at http://www.ifpri.org. It

---

[13] This short guide is meant as a starting point from which special interests can then be pursued. Web-addresses were correct at the time of writing.

provides information and the possibility to download documents in particular on the linkages between HIV/AIDS, food security and nutrition. Related to IFPRI is RENEWAL, the Regional Network on HIV/AIDS, Rural Livelihoods and Food Security in sub-Saharan Africa, which brings together national networks of agricultural institutions; public, private, nongovernmental and farmer organisations; and partners working on AIDS and health issues at http://www.ifpri.org/renewal/index.htm.

Lastly, the website of the International Fund for Agricultural Development (IFAD) at http://www.ifad.org can be searched for literature on HIV/AIDS and a number of documents linking the epidemic to poverty and development in general and agriculture in particular can be accessed.

In addition, a number of countries have set up their own websites which provide a guide to the status of the epidemic and its impact - one of the best examples is the comprehensive website of the Uganda AIDS Commission at http://www.aidsuganda.org/aids/index.htm.

Other sites - partly with a focus on Africa - with the possibility to search for and access documents on HIV/AIDS and wider development issues include the Support for Analysis and Research in Africa (SARA) site at http://sara.aed.org, and the site of the International AIDS Economics Network (IAEN) at http://www.iaen.org.

For a literature search on HIV/AIDS related issues, the following sites are useful:
The ELDIS Gateway to Development Information database, in particular the HIV/AIDS Resource Guide at
http://www.eldis.org/hivaids/index.htm;
the library database of the African Studies Centre in Leiden, in particular the dossier HIV/AIDS in Africa at
http://asc.leidenuniv.nl/library/webdossiers/dossierhivaids.htm; and
the database of the Ethiopia AIDS Resource Centre to be accessed at
http://www.etharc.org/InternetSearch/IntermediateSearch/IntMatlSearch.cfm

Lastly, concerning data on the status of the epidemic, the United States Census Bureau provides probably the most comprehensive, detailed and regularly updated picture of the epidemic worldwide. Wherever available, data is disaggregated into urban and rural datasets, the latter of particular importance when looking at HIV/AIDS and smallholder agriculture. The database can be accessed at http://www.census.gov/ipc/www/hivaidsn.html.

www.ingramcontent.com/pod-product-compliance
Lightning Source LLC
Chambersburg PA
CBHW081550220326
41598CB00036B/6632